THE STRANGE MEDICAL SAGA OF HOWARD HUGHES

By

Forest Tennant

AF869878

Published by the
Tennant Foundation
West Covina, California

Copyright© 2021 Tennant Foundation

Second Edition

All rights reserved. This book or any portion thereof may not be reproduced or used in any manner whatsoever without the express written permission of the publisher except for the use of brief quotations in a book review or scholarly journal.

ISBN: 9781955934091
Library of Congress Control Number: 2021912855

Ordering Information:

Special discounts are available on quantity purchases by corporations, associations, educators, and others. For details, contact the publisher at the below listed address.

U.S. trade bookstores and wholesalers: Please contact Nancy Kriskovich Tel: (406)249-2002;
or email snkriskovich@gmail.com
Medical Research and Education Project
c/o Nancy Kriskovich
14 Hidden River Lane
Bigfork, MT 59911

All proceeds from the sale of this book will go to the Medical Research and Education Project sponsored by the TENNANT FOUNDATION.
336 ½ S. GLENDORA AVENUE
WEST COVINA, CA 91790-3060
A 501(c)(3) Non-profit Organization

BOARD OF DIRECTORS

Chairperson: Jerry Muszynski
President: Forest Tennant
Vice President: Miriam Tennant
Secretary: Kathy Clark
Treasurer: James Hetzel

BOARD MEMBERS

Doran Barnes
Steve Castillo
Sander De Wildt
Don Scheliga
Vicki Scheliga
Tony Song
Ken Yoho

MEDICAL RESEARCH AND EDUCATION COMMITTEE

Chairperson: Ingrid Hollis
Terry Anderson
Lynn Ashcraft
Donna Corley
Lloyd Costello, MD
K. Scott Guess, Pharm D
Ryle Holder, Pharm D
Adam Hy, DO
Nancy Kriskovich
Denise Molohon
Kristen Ogden
Martin J. Porcelli, DO, PhD
Rhonda Posey
Tina Schofield
ReAnn S. Rothwell-Kingsland
Gary Snook

DEDICATION

This book is dedicated to the members of the Tennant Foundation Medical Research and Education Committee who tirelessly and with great dedication produce the education materials and operate the websites for the medical disorders that are targets of our research:

- Arachnoiditis
- Intractable Pain Syndrome

ACKNOWLEDGMENTS

This book could not have been researched and written without the technical assistance of Becky and Tom Marino and Nancy Kriskovich. Priscilla Sellers provided most helpful suggestions for this book.

Table of Contents

AUTHOR'S NOTE

Why did I write this book about the medical saga of Howard Hughes (HH)? The short answer is that the story of HH is part of history and needs to be recorded. The other is that no one else has the information I have from being personally involved in the case, along with the clinical experience to be able to write it. This book is more than just a history of HH. Any serious medical practitioner can learn a lot from HH. What is more, anyone who suffers from one of HH's three major medical conditions will find his saga most instructive.

About two years after HH died the federal government approached me and asked that I be a medical consultant on the case. My task was to research the medical history of HH and give an opinion as to whether his physicians had illegally supplied HH with narcotics (today called opioids). In 1978 I was one of very few physicians in the United States who was researching opioid addiction and treating severe chronic pain. My area of expertise was determining who was an addict and who was a legitimate pain patient that needed opioids for therapeutic purposes. My interest in these issues began when I served as a US Army physician between 1968 and 1972. It was during this time that our soldiers in Vietnam and Germany first began to use opioids and other abusable drugs. I treated many of the addicted soldiers and I vividly recall prescribing my first dose of methadone to withdraw an Army soldier addicted to opium. My formal, advanced medical training was in internal medicine at the Universities of Louisville and Texas following graduation from the Kansas Medical School. As an internist I had certainly become aware of the need for opioids in persons who suffered from tuberculosis, cancer, or autoimmune disease. Following my active duty in the Army, in 1972, I transferred to the US Public Health Service as an academic, post-doctoral fellow at the UCLA School of Public Health. My purpose was to obtain a masters and second doctoral degree so I could carry on research into the treatment of addiction and severe pain as I believed these were emerging and serious public health problems. In 1975 I set up a clinical research and treatment clinic in West Covina 40 miles across town from the UCLA campus. I started methadone and detoxification programs for heroin addicts and began to determine which severe pain patients needed opioids for painful conditions. By 1978, when the government asked for help, I knew enough to distinguish an opioid addict from a pain patient needing opioids for control of pain. Other avenues of my research at that time were to develop urine testing to detect drugs of abuse. A fact that has long-since been forgotten is that it was my personal research laboratory in which urine testing for the Los Angeles Dodgers and National Football League were initially performed. Also, at that time my research led to some of the detoxification and treatment techniques for alcohol, heroin, and cocaine dependence that are in use today. Palliative and end-of-life care for intractable pain patients was initiated.

To assist my investigation, the government gave me all the medically related documents that they were able to scrounge up from the secret and mysterious life of HH. They included Hughes' autopsy report, post-mortem toxicology analysis, birth certificate, death certificate, a 1958 memo written by Hughes involving medication acquisition, and a daily log of Hughes activities kept by his aides and dated October 31, 1971 through July 1, 1973. I was also given x-rays of HH's arms taken at the time of autopsy. Many of these documents are published in the appendix of this book to ensure that they will be available to future scholars and writers.

I compiled a report in September 1978 for the government that is published here, verbatim, as I was able to ascertain the cause of his death and the reason for his codeine use. This report became a public document later that year when it was presented in the federal trial involving Dr. Wilbur Thain, HH's last personal physician. Prior to the trial, the US Government and I believed Dr. Thain had illegally prescribed and administered codeine to HH as no medical records or other evidence was available to suggest otherwise. In the trial, however, medical records and testimony was produced so that Dr. Thain earned an acquittal by the jury.

My initial 1978 research into HH's medical saga determined that he began the use of codeine compound just after his 1946 plane crash in an experimental reconnaissance plane known as the XF-11. Codeine compound at that time contained a chemical called phenacetin which, if taken over a long period, can cause kidney failure which is the cause of HH's death listed on his death certificate.

I have chosen to write the medical saga of HH for some specific personal reasons. I am quite sure I am the only person alive who had the privilege to personally know and have a physician-to-physician visit with the last three of HH's personal physicians (Lawrence Chaffin, Norman Crane, Wilbur Thain). These visits gave me some insight into the reasons behind many seemingly bizarre happenings that occurred in the life of HH. These physicians were quite prominent and successful, as HH had the means to hire the best physicians at that time. Unfortunately, their involvement with HH unfairly tarnished their reputations. All three carried the opinion that HH was exceedingly difficult to treat as he was resistant to almost any therapeutic suggestion. They also recognized that he had medical conditions that were strange and unknown to them. Indeed, during the time of HH's life he had three major medical conditions that were neither well recognized nor understood: (1) obsessive compulsive disorder (OCD), (2) traumatic brain injury (TBI), and (3) intractable pain syndrome (IPS). In fact, these three conditions have only been understood well enough in recent years to make this book possible. Sad to say, HH did not have access to today's treatment of these conditions, or his life and saga would undoubtedly have been much different.

During the time I prepared my report for the government and testified in the Thain trial, a fair amount of publicity identified me as "the expert" on HH's medical conditions. Consequently, many persons have sought me out over the past 40 years to give me information about HH. In addition, a few close patients and colleagues knew of my interest in HH and that I remained mystified about his condition. Over the 40 years I have often been quoted in articles and have received three gifts which I make note of here. One is a piece of HH's Hercules Flying Boat known popularly as the Spruce Goose that fell off when it was moved from Long Beach, California to McMinnville, Oregon on February 27, 1992. Another is the picture which is on the cover and reputed to be Howard Hughes standing on a plane with writing that indicates it is the "Spirit of Saint Louis." It was flown by Charles Lindbergh to Paris in 1927. The picture was left in Hughes Hollywood offices by Noah Dietrich when he left the company on May 12, 1957. The exact date, location, and purpose of the picture is unknown except that HH was active in financing and promoting experimental aircraft between 1926 and 1935. A young man gave it to me who injured his neck in a serious accident in the 1980's. He was in terrible pain, disabled, and never could afford an x-ray of his neck. After his injury he made a living hustling old movie posters and paraphernalia that he scrounged and hustled in Hollywood. Hence, he came upon this picture. Over 30 years he paid me for his care by giving me movie posters and what appears to be a rare HH picture. The third thing I consider a gift is a letter sent to me on September 4, 2007 from Arelo Sederberg, who was the spokesman for HH's Summa Corporation, when HH died. The letter is reprinted verbatim in the chapter "Medical Facts Erase Some Myths." It elegantly summarizes much of the life and accomplishments of HH in a few words. Few publications have had much good to say about HH, but Arelo handily gives credit where it is due.

Several excellent investigative books about HH have been written by some of America's best journalists. The ones I have used for this book are referenced in the "Special Bibliography." I have interwoven HH's medical history into the vignettes, stories, and incidents that are vividly and succinctly described in one or more of the books. Simply stated, I could not have written this book had the books written in the "Special Bibliography" not laid a historic foundation that allowed medical information to be added.

This book has been written with the essential aid of the "Medical Research and Education Committee" of the Tennant Foundation. They are a most dedicated, fun group, and some of the members have one or more of the medical disorders that afflicted HH. This book is dedicated to them.

PROLOGUE

Howard Hughes (HH) was born an engineering and mechanical genius in 1905. He was also born into great wealth and inherited two diseases: obsessive compulsive disorder (OCD) and partial deafness that would plague his entire life of 70 years. Between his wealth and genius, he was able to accomplish feats in aviation and entertainment that have endured and benefitted society for over a century. Today's public knows Howard primarily for his OCD and his intense phobia of germs that were highlighted in the movie, "The Aviator." In the last century it was different. The public knew him for his aviation accomplishments, film making, romantic escapades with Hollywood starlets, and political machinations. Many of his behaviors and actions were quite repulsive, and there is little question they have over shadowed and obscured his many positive contributions to society.

Beginning in the mid 1950's at about age 55, he essentially disappeared from public life and began to lead a secretive, reclusive existence. So invisible was HH that a common cliché in the latter part of his life was, "We've heard about him but have never seen him." He died a mysterious death on April 5, 1976 while on a plane traveling from Acapulco, Mexico to Houston, Texas. The mystery became even more strange when Methodist Hospital in Houston performed an autopsy on April 6, 1976 and his estranged family quickly buried him on April 7, 1976. The cause of death announced by Methodist Hospital was kidney failure. No pictures of HH were taken and no other history or medical facts were given. Media reports expressed shock at his mysterious death and rapid burial which took place within 48 hours after he died. Unexpectedly, on April 10, 1976, three days after he was buried in the family plot at Glenwood Cemetery in Houston, a toxicologic analysis of his blood and body fluids surfaced which showed the presence of a significant amount of the narcotic (now called opioid), codeine. Methodist Hospital provided no explanation for this unexpected finding. The medical examiner (coroner), Dr. Joseph A. Jachimczyk, however, explained codeine's presence this way, "There's no question the man was in pain."

Surprisingly, HH had not left a will. On April 10, 1976, it was clear that the richest man in the world died mysteriously with an opioid in his blood and without a will. Immediately all sorts of conspiracy theories of murder, forced addiction, medical neglect, and claims to his estate hit the media. Investigations, lawsuits, and books began "in mass." Within 18 months two of the physicians, Dr. Norman Crane and Dr. Wilbur Thain, who had cared for HH in the last few years of his life, were indicted on federal charges of illegally prescribing and administering narcotic drugs to HH. These indictments led to the hiring of this author by the Federal Government, and they initiated the beginning of a serious investigation into the medical saga of HH.

The first major findings at HH's autopsy were that the cause of his death was kidney failure from phenacetin, an ingredient in codeine formulations at that time in history. The use of codeine was initiated to treat his pain after he sustained severe injuries in a July 7, 1946 air crash of the experimental reconnaissance plane, XF-11. HH was so seriously injured in the crash that he was lucky to survive. Due to many burns and injuries sustained in the crash, he required codeine for pain control for the remaining 30 years of his life. He developed a condition we now call the Intractable Pain Syndrome (IPS) which is constant, incurable pain that produces cardiovascular and endocrine complications.

To complicate HH's medical history, he not only had OCD and partial deafness, but also sustained multiple episodes of head trauma between 1929 and 1951. In today's terminology it is referred to as "Traumatic Brain Injury" (TBI). Only very recently has medical science understood the serious ramifications of the three major medical disorders that plagued HH: (1) obsessive compulsive disorder (OCD), (2) traumatic brain injury (TBI), and (3) intractable pain syndrome (IPS). Many of the bizarre behavioral actions and traits of HH ranging from reclusiveness to germ phobia can be explained by his medical conditions. Many myths and questions surrounding his life such as a conspiracy to murder him with codeine are either debunked or answered now that his medical history and disorders are fully understood. From a purely medical viewpoint, HH is a treasure trove of medical education. He was a once-in-a-lifetime case. It is highly doubtful that we will ever again see a combination of such fascinating and personal details in one person: the richest man in the world who was a mechanical genius and who simultaneously suffered from OCD, TBI, and IPS.

1. Introduction

The front page of the New York Times on April 6, 1976 featured this headline: "Howard Hughes (HH) Dies at 70 on Flight to Texas Hospital" with the sub-headline, "Billionaire was Flying from Acapulco with Undisclosed Illness." Along with this headline was a picture of HH sporting a fedora hat and a moustache. This was one of the last pictures of HH which was taken in the early 1950's. The headline telling the public that HH had died was shocking in 1976, as the once wildly famous billionaire, playboy tycoon, Hollywood movie mogul, and aviation innovator had been out of public view for so many years that many thought he was already dead. The truth was that Hughes had entered a phantom-like reclusive lifestyle in 1966 when, at the age of 61, he moved into the top floor of the Desert Inn in Las Vegas and had not been heard from since. He left Las Vegas for the Bahamas on Thanksgiving Eve in 1970 and had not returned to the United States since that time. During these six years he lived in luxury hotels in different countries and was very much alive and was still actively involved in his business endeavors.

The flight on which he died was headed to Methodist Hospital in Houston to obtain emergency medical care for an ailment that was unknown to his doctors. He died 30 minutes before arrival at the hospital. Methodist Hospital, unintentionally, fostered the mystery of HH. Their only press release said that HH was originally on his way to get medical treatment at their institution but died before he arrived. The hospital performed an autopsy and merely said he died of kidney failure. To help silence all medical facts about this mysterious man, his estranged family, saw to it that he was buried within 48 hours after his plane landed in Houston. There were no pictures taken of HH, and neither the doctors who cared for him late in his life nor those who performed his autopsy granted interviews. Then an unexpected event occurred three days after his burial. Blood and other body fluids that had been taken during his autopsy and sent to an outside specialty laboratory for what is called a toxicology analysis, reported their findings on April 10, 1976. It showed significant levels of the narcotic (hereafter called opioid) codeine, in his blood, bile, urine, liver, and stomach.

The public was shocked and stupefied. By April 11, just 6 days after he died, the public only knew that a famous, billionaire recluse of the 20th century had died of kidney disease and had codeine in his body fluids. Concern over any "why and in what manner" involving his medical issues and cause of death, however, consumed the news for only a few days. The big public interest and concern about HH turned to his millions and who was going to inherit them. HH did not leave a will, so the claims and lawsuits over his will and inheritance started before his graveside flowers began to wilt. Journalists, writers, and movie makers realized the public was enamored with the life of HH. Money, sex, Hollywood, and politics always made a far better story than why the tubules in his kidneys stopped working. An uncounted number of books, shows, and writings began and have continued into recent years. Before 1976, the year of his death, was over, enterprising, and esteemed writers managed to grab some of HH's aides and pump out all sorts of stories. Two bestselling books, one called, "Howard Hughes: The Hidden Years," and the other "The Hughes Papers" were published within six months after he died.

The finding of codeine in HH's blood fueled a different but mysterious avenue of intrigue and inquiry other than money, women, and politics. Since codeine is an opioid and he died of kidney failure, the reasoning was that there must be conspiracy or hanky-panky to explain this combination. Theories started. Could he have been murdered with codeine? Was he forcibly addicted to codeine to control his financial empire? Was he deprived of medical care to force an early death? No wonder that government prosecutors piled on with a frenzy of lawsuits and investigations. While most of the government prosecutors went after HH's money, some believed that codeine in his body fluids meant that a crime had been committed, so they wanted to track down the facts.

The latter is where I came in. After HH died I was as intrigued and fascinated with HH as anyone else. I, for one, was not sure exactly what to make of the whole HH story. After all, I had heard of him but did not have a clue as to what he looked like or even how he had made his money. Then, out of the blue, in the summer of 1978, I received a telephone call from the Federal Drug Enforcement Agency. Federal prosecutors believed that HH was either murdered with codeine or that his doctors, in conjunction with Summa Corporation executives, kept HH addicted to control his money and empire or facilitate an early death by medical neglect. The government wanted me to investigate and analyze the few documents they had scrounged about HH relative to his secretive medical condition and codeine use. They believed that HH's personal physicians and aides had illegally suppled HH with codeine for nefarious purposes. My task was to figure out what medically happened, why he died, prepare a written analysis, and testify in court if I believed HH's physicians had illegally prescribed and administered codeine and other drugs to HH. The challenge to understand the medical history of such an icon was something I could not turn down. In 1978 I began my search and analysis for the medical facts and understanding of a strange, one-of-a-kind, medical saga. This book relates an amazing and bizarre story of HH as it unfolds through the lens of my medical investigations. It is a tale that you could not possibly make up in your wildest imagination. Truth and history are ofttimes stranger than fiction! My longtime search has uncovered a strange medical saga that is educational history at its best and one for the ages.

2. Humble Beginnings – 1905-1925

"A Mechanical Genius is Born"

The saga begins on December 24, 1905 in Humble, Texas. He was born to Allene and Howard Hughes, Sr with the name Howard Robard Hughes, Jr. Today, Humble is a quiet, Houston suburb of slightly over 15,000 people. In 1905, however, it became an oil boomtown with it being the biggest producing field in Texas. The town was named after Pleasant Smith Humble who settled there, around 1889 to primarily harvest timber for railroad ties. Between 1889 and 1904 it was a country conclave with farms and sawmills, but in 1904 a man named CE Barrett drilled for oil and hit a small production site on an area called Moonshine Hill. A few months later, on January 7, 1905 he brought in a second oil producing well called the "Beaty Well" yielding 8500 barrels a day. This set off the boom with the population growing from a village of about 700 to 20,000 within two years. Humble became the home of the Humble Oil and Refining Company that was the predecessor of Exxon. HH's father became Humble's greatest asset. He invented the oil drilling bit with 166 cutting edges that allowed drilling into rock formations and the extraction of oil and gas. Howard, Sr. patented the drill bit but never sold it. He formed the Hughes Tool Company to produce the bit. He only rented out the drill bit which produced the millions of dollars that launched the life and activities of HH. Put another way, the world can thank a brilliant father, drill bit, and Humble, Texas for the amazing, awesome life of HH. The invention of the drill bit was one of the great advances of the 20th century. It allowed oil drilling through hard rock and sand so oil could come to the surface. This single invention has given us the ability to drive our cars and heat our homes, among all the other necessities that petroleum products have given to the development of modern society. HH was right to call his father the "smartest man I ever met."

The birth of HH was the foundation of his medical saga. He was born with two genetic health issues that would plague him through the 70 years of his life. First, he had partial deafness. He had a long family history of deafness. This undoubtedly had something to do with his social aloofness, shyness, and avoidance of crowds. Equally if not even more serious was the fact that he inherited from his mother a rare disease now known as obsessive-compulsive disorder (OCD). HH had a bizarre childhood primarily because his mother had a severe form of OCD. Consequently, he had multiple medical and psychologic events in his childhood and teenage years that influenced his medical conditions later in life. The relationship between HH and his mother was hardly that of a normal mother-son relationship. From infancy HH often slept in his mother's room on a small trundle bed. At the least hint of a fever or the slightest sign of a rash, physicians were rushed to the house, no matter what hour. Each morning and evening, Allene, ordered her son to be naked and "stand still Howard." She checked his teeth, ears, genitals, elbows, and kneecaps. Then she checked the contents of his toilet. "Now you can flush" she would tell him. She saw to it that he had cod liver oil and Russian mineral oil in the morning and used Epsom salts in the evening. Each day she bathed him from head-to-toe using strong lye soap.

Howard's mother also did her best to shield him from the other boys in town. No wonder. Humble, in the early part of the last century, was an oil boom town. Such towns were a wild setting with money, fights, drunkenness, and promiscuity. In fact,

Howard's father was promiscuous and left his wife at home for long periods as he traveled to market his drill bit. He spent a lot of time in Southern California since, like Houston, it was beginning to find oil and needed the Hughes oil bit. Howard, Sr. spent a lot of time with the Hollywood crowd and its' "all too eager women." Howard, Jr. traveled with his father to Hollywood on a few occasions and in his teenage years attended Thatcher High in Ojai and some classes at Caltech in Pasadena.

Despite the obsessions his mother had about germs and Howard's health, she appeared to do her best to bring him up to be a disciplined and thoughtful person. In October 1906 Howard, Sr., and his wife, Allene, traveled with baby Howard to Keokuk, Iowa to visit Howard, Sr.'s parents. While there, they had baby Howard baptized into the Episcopal faith, officiated by the Reverend R.C. McIlwain. Back home in Humble, his mother had him attend church and Sunday School. At age 10 he was crowned "king" of the Christ Church Cathedral's, May Fete, an annual spring rite staged for the children of the elite congregation. There were a lot of children in Humble, but Howard did not socialize much with them. He had, however, a close friend his age, Dudley C. Sharp, whose father was the partner of Howard, Sr. Dudley was best man at HH's wedding to Ella Rice in 1925.

Howard's parents, especially his mother, did not want HH to be exposed to the social and community life of a boom town. There is no record of HH belonging to Cub or Boy Scouts, 4-H, team sports, or bands. In 1920, at the age of 14, he was sent to Boston to attend Fessenden School in West Newton, Massachusetts. Founded in 1903, the school was for sons of wealthy parents who were counting on the school to polish their boys into suitable Ivy League material. Howard studied hard and was cited for "outstanding industry and attention to studies." At the school he became interested and excelled at golf. He remained at Fessenden for about a year. His father then arranged to enroll him at the prestigious, private Thatcher School in Ojai, CA, because the family was spending a lot of time in Los Angeles since Southern California had discovered oil and needed the Hughes drill bit.

Health issues and his medical saga began to surface in HH's childhood which were largely unknown until after HH's death. After his death in 1976, Will Lummis, a member of the Hughes family, took over reins of HH's company, the Summa Corporation. To help defend against lawsuits over the inheritance of HH, he hired psychologist Raymond D. Fowler, Jr, PhD and psychiatrist, John Chappell, MD to do what was called a "psychologic autopsy" on HH. While this "autopsy" was mainly drafted to excuse HH and the Summa Corporation from any legal liability or sharing of inheritance, they examined HH's childhood.

Dr. Fowler and Chapelle's investigation and report provides a great understanding of HH's early medical issues. By age ten Drs. Fowler and Chapelle, labeled HH a "uniquely talented hypochondriac." He apparently had a versatile repertoire of ailments including chills and episodes of malaise that would stump physicians. Modern psychoanalysts would likely label HH an "avoider," a person who uses psychosomatic illness to escape from life. Howard learned early on that he could get what he wanted by feigning illness.

The most notable episode of feigned or psychologic illness occurred in April 1920 when HH was 15 years old. He suddenly developed paralysis of his legs and could not walk. At the onset of the paralysis episode, he was found one morning in his bedroom groaning and delirious. Doctors found no evidence of a real disease as he had no fever, swelling, rash, or abnormalities in his blood. After about eight weeks of paralysis that required a wheelchair for ambulation, he suddenly recovered. Despite consultation with several prominent physicians, no specific medical cause of this paralytic episode was determined. A doctor, H.T.

Chickering, a pioneer in polio research, suspected that Howard was feigning illness and labeled the cause "hysterical paralysis."

Little has been recorded about the seriousness of HH's genetic deafness. Exactly how serious it was or if it was present in early childhood is not precisely known. Deafness can have a serious impact on one's ability to socialize and communicate. It may have played a role in the development of his many medical symptoms before the age of ten, or even later in life. HH's deafness either worsened or emerged during his teenage years. HH at one point in his late teenage years stated that his hearing was damaged while swimming. In later life he told Katherine Hepburn and Faith Domergue that his deafness was triggered and worsened in an auto accident. Interestingly, nothing has been recorded as to "how deaf" he was or if HH used it to avoid issues or verbal input. He never wore a hearing aid and his physicians stated that his deafness was a barrier to communication and the administration of medical care. Interestingly, a comment by a silent film star, Eleanor Boardman, somewhat clarifies his deafness. In the early 1920's Hollywood, like Humble, had become a boom town, but the driving force was silent film making rather than oil. Howard, Sr's brother, Rupert Hughes, was a major producer of silent films. It is poorly appreciated or recognized that Uncle Rupert was the original connection and attraction of HH's desire to make films. One of the premier social and business gatherings of Hollywood insiders during the "Roaring 20's" was a Sunday brunch put on by Rupert. One Sunday Howard, Jr. accompanied his father to one of the brunches. There he met Eleanor Boardman who was a beautiful, 23-year-old, hazel eyed actress starring in the silent film "Souls for Sale," a movie being directed by Rupert. Young Howard became infatuated with her and wanted to date her. The feeling was not mutual, and Eleanor told Howard Sr. in rejecting him that he was," very unattractive, very shy, hard of hearing, and difficult." While Ms. Boardman's life and film endeavors are irrelevant to this book, her comment about HH being "hard of hearing" is medically important. Good hearing is essential to communication and socialization. This defect combined with OCD clearly put some barriers in place that HH had to overcome to be successful.

During his childhood and teenage years his superior, native intelligence and mechanical prowess began to emerge along with his hypochondria and deafness. In 1916 at the age of 11, he built, operated, and even licensed a ham radio set. A year later he built a motorized bicycle with parts from one of his father's steam engines. At age 14 he learned to fly an airplane and his father purchased a Stutz Bearcat automobile for him. He took it apart and reassembled it within a month. In summary, by HH's teenage years it was clear that he was some sort of mechanical and engineering genius with a hypochondriacal personality.

In 1922 at age 17, his mother, Allene, died at age 39 of an ectopic pregnancy. Likely the loss of his wife put undue stress onto Howard, Sr. as he died from a heart attack within 24 months after her death at the age of 54. The deaths of both parents by the time one is 19 years of age would, of course, be a life-altering shock for anyone. Howard, Jr. was obviously remorseful, but he knew he had to act fast and aggressively to inherit and save the Hughes Tool Company. HH sought and was legally declared an emancipated minor, and he inherited about 75% of Hughes Tool Co., which was worth about $5 million in 1924. To be declared an emancipated minor he had to convince the court in Houston that he could run the Hughes Tool Company.

At the time of his father's death, in 1929, he was attending Rice University. There he met and eventually married, Ella Botts Rice on June 1, 1925. She was a grandniece of William Marsh Rice who founded Rice Institute. Two nights before his wedding to Ella Rice, HH signed a will that was designed to protect his inheritance. He was particularly concerned about community property laws that would give the burgeoning Hughes Tool Company to the relatives of Ella. He proceeded to give $75,000 to his Aunt Janet Houston and $1000 and the family home to his aunt, Annette Lumas. He designated $500,000 in "first class, high grade securities to my wife, Ella Rice Hughes." Surprisingly, he wanted the rest of his estate to go to the establishment of the "Howard P. Hughes Medical Research Laboratories," to be created "as soon after my death as practicable." At that time, he charged the research effort with "scientific research for discovery and development of antitoxins and specific remedies for the cure and prevention of dangerous diseases." It is somewhat interesting that HH wanted to form a medical research institute. He maintained this desire throughout life and formed the Howard Hughes Medical Institute in 1953. It is very possible that his keen interest in medical research was based on his own infirmities and his medical interest may have led to some self-help measures that allowed him to live 70 years despite his horrific, medical conditions. For example, it is known that he became a great fan of vitamins and minerals at some point in his life. This author is unable to verify this, but I have been informed by some medical colleagues that he asked nutritionists at Harvard, at some point in the 1950's or 1960's, to make him a special vitamin-herbal preparation.

His Humble beginnings ended in 1925 at age 20. In the fall of that year, he took his wife Ella and moved to Los Angeles. So, with a business, worth millions, and a wife, he, at the ripe old age of 20, packed his bags and moved west with a plan and vision to associate with Uncle Rupert and make films in the new silent screen industry.

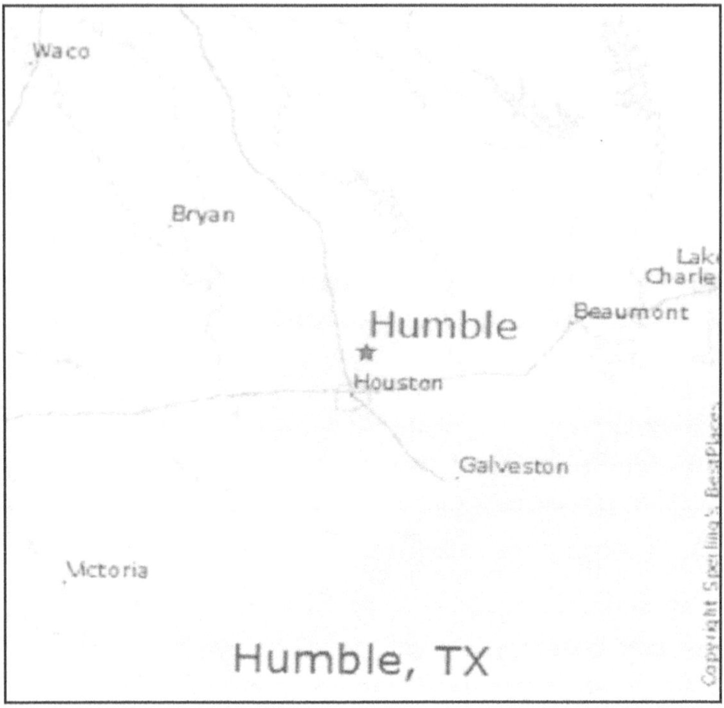

Humble, Texas was an oil boomtown in the early 1900's

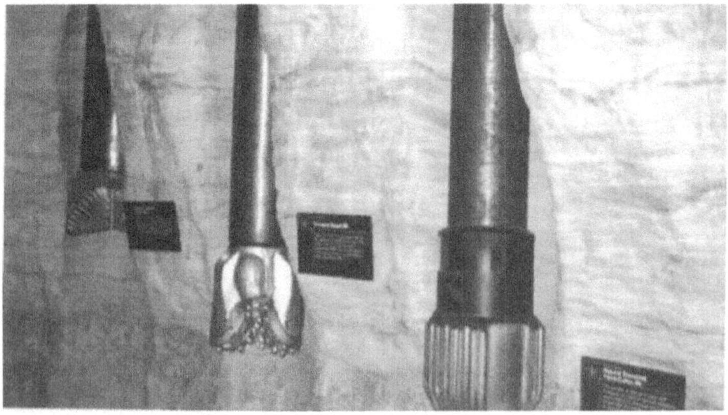

The Hughes oil drill bit would drill through packed sand and rock.

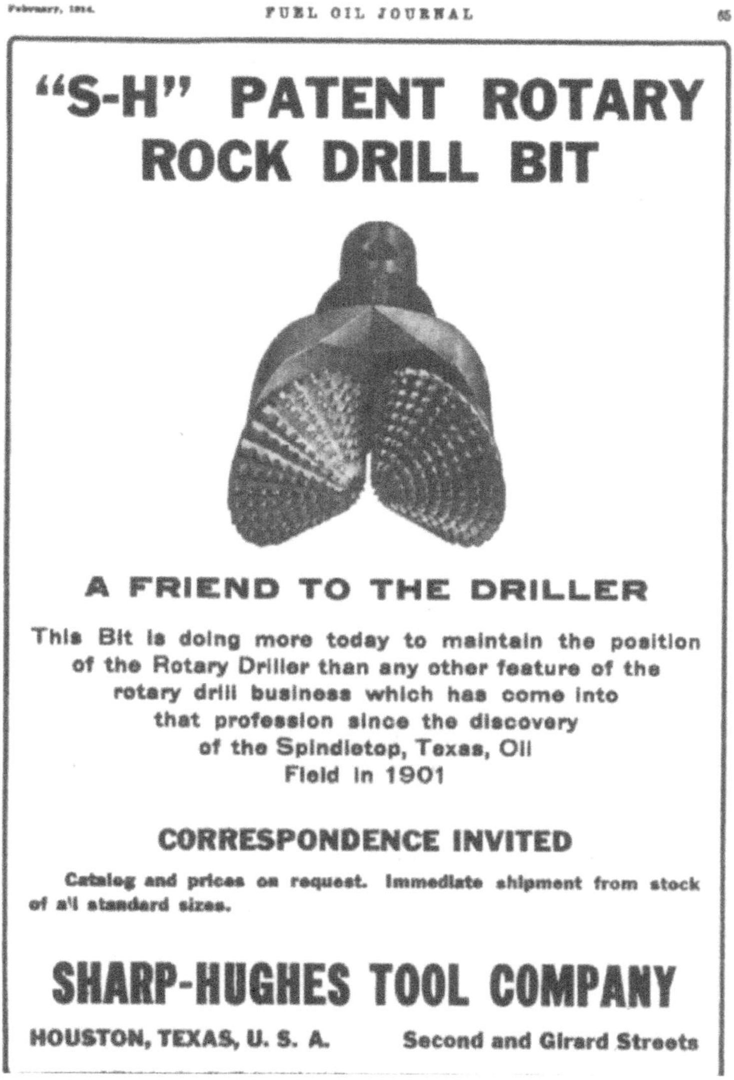

Advertisement for the Hughes Tool Bit-1914

3. Bad Health Erupts in Hollywood 1925-1932

"A Tragic Plane Crash"

In the fall of 1925 Hughes, at age 20, and his new wife, Ella, took up residence at the Ambassador Hotel in Los Angeles (LA). The Ambassador was west of downtown LA and close to Hollywood. HH had moved to Hollywood with a desire to make silent films. His Uncle Rupert was an elite producer and he had previously visited the Goldwyn Studios in Culver City. Hughes was fascinated as he watched silent movies being made. There are no reports of any serious health issues or peculiar behaviors attributed to Hughes after his paralysis recovery at about age 15 and his move to Los Angeles. He also remained in apparent good health for about three more years until he started filming Hell's Angels in 1928.

Before the end of 1925, Hughes went right to work in establishing his business operations including oversight of the tool company and a corporate move to establish his film making operation. He amended one of the tool company subsidiaries, the Caddo Rock Drill Bit Company of Louisiana, which allowed it to not only lease drill bits but make films. Caddo thus became the vehicle for his early film making. HH rented office space in the Taft Building at Hollywood and Vine that was a central location in the heart of movie-making land. He then hired Noah Dietrich (ND) in

November 1925 to oversee his Hollywood operations. HH continued to oversee the Tool Company. In summary by the end of 1925, at age 22, HH had married, moved to LA, opened an office, and hired an executive overseer of operations. He was ready to start his film-making career.

The hiring of ND was a profound and positive one as he not only astutely made millions for HH, but essentially cared for him as he later developed severe health issues. ND was a stocky, gruff-talking former accountant who was the perfect person for the job, as he was shrewd and ambitious. Even more important, he was tolerant and accepting of HH's medical issues as he had to step in to literally save his life on at least two occasions. ND was with HH for 32 years until May 12, 1957 when he was fired. In these decades ND closely partnered with HH to build his financial empire and even keep him alive by obtaining necessary medical care.

To firmly establish himself in LA and boost his film-making company, he and his wife, Ella, purchased a Spanish style home in 1926 for $135,000 that was located at 211 Muirfield Road in the ritzy Hancock Park section of town. Many movie people were settling in this area. The back of the house overlooked the Wilshire Country Club where Hughes regularly played golf. At one point in his early life, he had aspirations of becoming the "world's best golfer" but his overseeing of the Hughes Tool Company and film-making endeavors squashed any hopes to be a big name in the golf game. Albeit to say, however, he reputedly was a talented golfer who might just have made it big on the professional circuit.

For his first film venture, Hughes teamed up with Ralph Graves, an actor whom Hughes Sr. had once placed on the tool company's payroll. Graves had acquired a story called "Swell Hogan" that he was convinced would make a great movie. Hughes invested about sixty thousand dollars and let Graves do the rest. The finished product was apparently so bad that the movie was never released. On his next try, Hughes hired Marshall Neilan, an old friend of his father, to direct a comedy called "Everybody's Acting." Critics liked it and the film made a modest profit. Within three years Hughes and Dietrich went on to produce "Two Arabian Knights," "All Quiet on the Western Front," and "Of Mice and Men." Two Arabian Knights won an Academy Award in 1928, the second year of the awards. In three short years HH had clearly established himself as a player in the silent film industry.

Until 1928 HH had primarily been a financier of his films and his health was fundamentally good. Although there are some anecdotal reports of minor compulsive behaviors such as working long hours and repetitive actions such as multiple handwashing, there were no overt signs of extreme, unusual behaviors or poor judgement typical of severe OCD. This changed, however, when in 1927, at age 22, he decided he would not only finance but direct the movie "Hell's Angels." HH admired the deeds and valor of First World War airmen, and he wanted to make a gala movie about them. He initially hired two directors, but they could not get along, so HH took over directing the film on October 31, 1927 and began shooting indoor scenes at the Metropolitan Studios in Hollywood.

The decision to produce, finance and direct Hell's Angels was the start of his serious symptoms of OCD which are described in detail in following chapters. Suffice it to say, stress will accentuate, accelerate, and precipitate the symptoms of this disorder including illogical thinking, perfectionism, repetitive tasks, inadequate diet, hygiene, and insomnia. Although the filming of Hell's Angels was a great success and propelled his movie making reputation, it was the start of serious health issues that could have been prevented.

HH's OCD was evident in how he made the film. His directing led to the deaths of three of the pilots who died in fiery accidents during the filming. Hughes wanted the aerial scenes in the movie to be realistic, but this compulsion possibly caused the three deaths. To accomplish realism HH wanted actual First World War fighter planes. For months, his scouts toured Europe rounding up relics from the war. Among them were famous planes that went by the names Spads, Sopwith Camels, and Fokkers. In all he acquired or leased 87 vintage planes. He spent about $500,000 on aircraft. To fly them he hired World War I aces like Roscoe Turner and noted daredevil pilots.

The evidence that OCD was behind some decisions in making Hell's Angels was that he constantly wanted repetition of scenes to achieve "perfection." Observers were often amazed because the same scene shot multiple times was senseless since the view never really changed. His final selection of scenes was totally arbitrary and without rationale. To be realistic, on one occasion he wanted clouds in the sky, so he had to shoot some scenes in Oakland because LA did not have enough clouds.

HH wanted an audience-grabbing scene in which a scout plane was to dive toward the ground but pull back up when it is just 200 feet above the ground. None of the professional flyers and stuntmen hired to fly in the film would take the assignment. A World War I ace and one of Hollywood's most daring and busiest stunt fliers, Paul Mantz, warned HH that the plane would crash if flown below 1000 feet. HH began his obstinate public, bad judgements by flying this plane. On January 29, 1928 HH attempted the stunt. As predicted by the pros, it crashed. Hughes crawled out of the aircraft and the movie set crew found him grimacing and leaning against the wall of a newly constructed movie set hanger. His clothes were tattered and bloody. He began babbling about his golf game and collapsed into unconsciousness. An ambulance rushed him to the Inglewood Hospital. Noah Dietrich rushed to the hospital, registered HH under an assumed name, and found the best doctors available including Dr. Vernon Mason.

He remained in a coma for three days. He inconceivably awoke on the third day and returned to the movie set on the fourth day after the crash. He required some minor facial surgery that took away the cleft in his chin. A piece of metal lodged in his skull. Dr. Mason met and cared for HH during this incident and became his personal physician for the following three decades.

Another major health issue occurred during the filming of Hell's Angels. On June 1, 1929, HH stumbled home from filming on the set and threw himself into bed without undressing. Several hours later the housekeeper found him at the edge of consciousness and believed he was dying. She contacted Noah Dietrich, who summoned Dr. Vernon Mason. Both Dietrich and Mason kept vigil for 48 hours. Dr. Mason diagnosed spinal meningitis. He believed HH might die as spinal meningitis was often fatal in 1929 since no antibiotics had yet been discovered. It is unknown what treatments may have been rendered, but HH lived. Despite the air crashes and deaths with this film, it was a huge success. Whether it did or did not make a profit has been a subject of debate. Regardless, it launched Jean Harlow as a female star and brought recognition to HH as an expert film producer. After Hell's Angels, HH was headline news, and his movies and love affairs with Hollywood starlets captured the imagination of the public for about the next twenty-five years.

A common manifestation of OCD is germaphobia. HH was terribly afflicted with this obsession. Typically, HH washed his hands repetitively, refused to shake hands, and sometimes covered objects to shield himself from imaginary, non-existent germs. Unfortunately, in 1932, he caught a real infection and went "ballistic."

Not long after Hell's Angels was filmed, shown, and declared a momentous financial and popular success, he contracted syphilis known as the "clap" in those days. It is unknown from whom he contracted it. Penicillin had not yet been invented, and the treatment, known as the "magic bullet," consisted of low levels of mercury and arsenic being periodically injected over five weeks. Syphilis then, as now, is primarily diagnosed by the presence of a sore or ulcer on the penis or vulva. It is called a "chancre." The causative germ, called a spirochete, is described as "secondary," or "tertiary" if it enters the blood or brain. Although syphilis almost always remains restricted to an ulcer on the sex organs, if it enters the brain, it causes a putty-like substance to be formed which is called a "gumma." Too much "gumma" may cause mental illness or dementia.

HH went into an acute germ phobia rage when he found out he had contracted syphilis. He summoned Noah Dietrich and four tool company staff to come to his house and remove and burn all clothing and bedding. In a non-logical, non-sensical manner, he stacked each clothing type in one pile. By the time staff and Dietrich arrived he had neat piles of sweaters, jackets, underwear, and shoes. HH commanded his aides put them in separate bags along with all bed linens. All these items were to be removed from the house and burned in the industrial kilns at the Long Beach Oil Fields. One aide wanted to know if he could keep one of HH's expensive jackets rather than just burn it. HH said yes but told the aide he would get syphilis if he wore it, and, furthermore, HH would not pay for his medical treatment. After his chancre healed, some of his physicians told him he had tertiary syphilis of the brain and that he would become sterile. These proved to be false statements as at least three women became pregnant by Hughes after his syphilis episode. After this episode he began to exhibit many germophobic manifestations, mental lapses, and some inappropriate decisions. Due to this emergence of bizarre behaviors both Noah Dietrich and Dr. Mason thought he may have developed tertiary syphilis. This proved not to be the case. What Dietrich and Mason were observing was a man who had severe symptomatic OCD complicated with a traumatic brain injury (TBI). At that time there was no concept of the development of mental symptoms following head trauma. Only many years later were the terms "Post-Concussion Syndrome" or "Traumatic Encephalopathy" used to describe the symptoms caused by head trauma. At some point in the mid-1930's his germophobic and bizarre behaviors were no longer attributed to tertiary syphilis since his OCD and TBI temporarily improved. Once tertiary syphilis developed in those days, symptoms did not improve but went on to cause blatant psychosis or dementia. Indeed, his autopsy 40 years later showed no evidence of the telltale gumma of tertiary syphilis.

HH's marriage did not last long. Shortly after arriving in LA, he began courting other women and leaving Ella alone for long periods. On October 1, 1928 Ella returned to Houston overstressed and exhausted. She was hospitalized at St. Joseph's Infirmary with the diagnosis of "ulcerative colitis," "nervous exhaustion," and "dehydration." The marriage was not destined to last. Ella Rice was a cultured, educated, and kind person who fit high society. HH was crude, insensitive, and uncultured. He was just the type of man who came out of the Texas oil patch in the early part of the 20th century. In mid-March 1929, she prepared a series of dinner receptions to unite Hollywood's various and disparate characters and egos. HH did not show up at all or late at best. This was apparently a last straw. For Ella, the marriage was over when Howard turned his back on her guests. She confessed to Noah Dietrich, "I tried. I really tried. But there's no point." The next day she left LA, returned to Houston, and filed for divorce which was finalized on December 9, 1929.

The extent of his TBI is incompletely known, but he began to experience some migraine headaches, memory lapses, and irrational acts, after the January 29, 1928 crash. Noah Dietrich stated his usual behaviors such as repetitions, hand washing, and fear of germs increased. Also, he began to experience periodic episodes of "heart racing" known technically as paroxysmal atrial tachycardia (PAT). HH apparently realized that his involvement with Hell's Angels had its punishments. In a rare interview in 1932 he confessed, "Making Hell's Angels by myself was my biggest mistake. It would have finished sooner and cost less. I had to worry about money, sign checks, hire pilots, get planes, cast everything, direct the whole thing. Trying to do the work of twelve men was just dumbness on my part. I learned by bitter experience that no one man can know everything." This statement does not explicitly say it, but one gets the impression that he may have believed his personal health and welfare may have been damaged as it certainly was. In summary, in his first six years in Hollywood, he suffered a TBI and had contracted two infections, meningitis, and syphilis. Also, his plane crash while filming "Hell's Angels" caused a TBI, so the combination of OCD and TBI affected him until death.

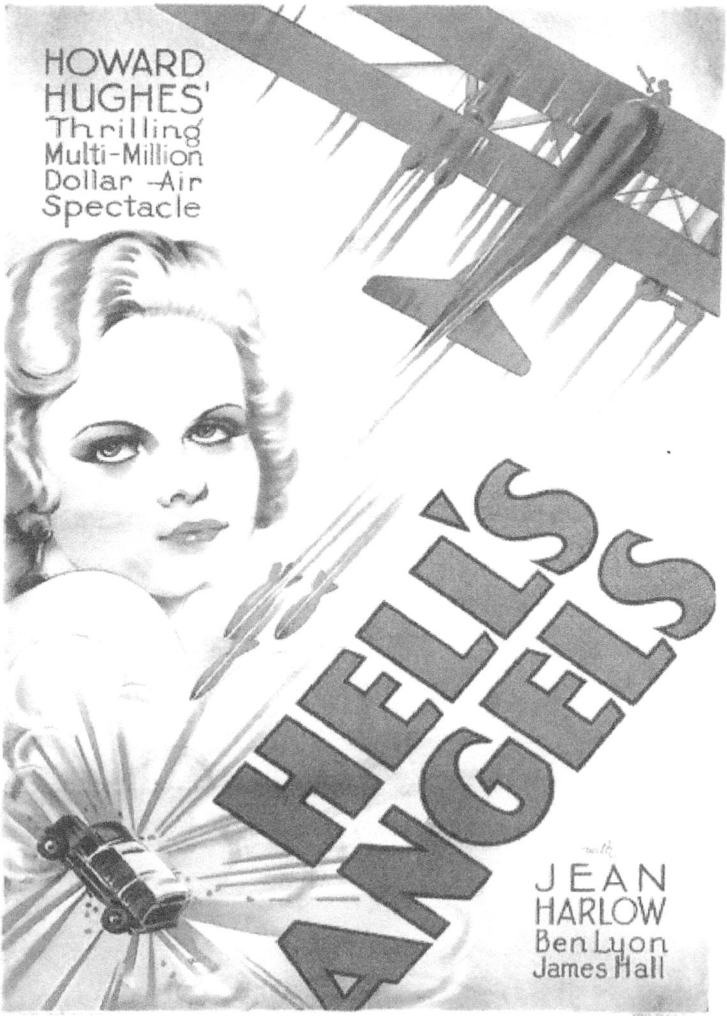

Movie poster advertising "Hells Angels." Hughes crashed in 1928, a scout plane and suffered his first concussion and traumatic brain injury. Afterward his obsessive-compulsive disorder (OCD) symptoms significantly emerged.

4. Hughes Crippling Disease: Obsessive-Compulsive Disorder – January 29, 1928-Forward

"Head Trauma Complication"

Ask anyone about HH and chances are they will say, "Oh yeah, he was that crazy guy who was always afraid of germs." Thanks to the movie, "Aviator," an entire mass of today's citizenry has negatively been introduced to a man who died over four decades ago. In fact, more people probably know more about HH's germ phobia than they do about any other aspect of his life including his women, money, politics, and movies, much less anything about his enduring accomplishments and gifts to society. OCD is characterized by obsessions which are recurrent, persistent, intrusive, or unwelcome thoughts, urges, or images and compulsions or repetitive behaviors or activities that the person feels forced to perform in response to an obsession. Unfortunately, OCD in those days and even today, is viewed by many inside and outside the medical profession to be a personality defect or voluntary malfunction that can be cured with "will power."[3,13,17] The first recognition that OCD was a serious genetic, medical condition didn't really begin to emerge until the 1950's.[38] For example, the 1956 Merck Manual, a physician's clinical handbook which began being periodically published in 1899, stated "the patient with an obsession or compulsion recognizes that his repetitive thoughts and acts are unreasonable, but he is unable to control them." Prior to this time OCD can hardly be found in medical publications.

Today OCD is identified as a genetic or hereditary disease of the central nervous system (CNS).[3,9,13,17,22,38] During the lifetime of HH, this disorder was not recognized as a disease but was usually called a "neurosis." The fact is that HH's OCD was the crippling disease that led to his other two major medical disorders, traumatic brain injury (TBI) and the intractable pain syndrome (IPS).

Beginning in his 20's after he moved to LA, he was observed to occasionally display a few minor compulsions and obsessions that are typical of OCD. In restaurants he requested unopened bottles of milk and always ordered the same meal. He wrapped the wheel of an airplane to form a barrier against germs. He often carried his own bar of soap to use in public restrooms. Typical with this disease there is the compulsive inclination to be quite driven, controlling, and perfectionistic. For example, he would repeatedly perform many tasks that were already completed and done well.

HH's obsessions and compulsions were harmless and earned him the title of "odd" or "eccentric" by his close acquaintances and "neurotic" by his doctors. As related in the last chapter, all this changed on January 29,1928. After he crashed a scout plane while filming "Hell's Angels," his head was traumatized, and he was in a coma for three days. A TBI or concussion will almost always change a person in some way. Why? Because the trauma causes inflammation, bleeding, and nerve tissue damage inside the brain. When brain tissue heals there is scarring. Scarred tissue is never the good, strong, vibrant tissue that was there before the damage.

A regular characteristic of brain trauma is to worsen any other affliction, mental or physical, that a person may have. For example, if you have a little tremor, you might start jerking or shaking. If you drink alcohol or smoke, your intake will shoot up. A person prone to occasional depression has it daily. A minor painful joint, nerve, or muscle may become disabled and paralytic. Simply put, TBI makes all other physical and mental infirmities worse including OCD. This happened to HH. Prior to his plane crash and coma, his OCD was a nuisance, but afterward it became a crippling, disorder that greatly impaired and periodically disabled him.

Beside an expert analysis of HH's childhood, insight into HH's OCD behavior and illness was analyzed and described by Drs. Raymond Fowler and John Chappell in their "psychologic autopsy."[10] To reach a conclusion these expert mental health professionals interviewed some of Hughes' former staff and evaluated newspaper reports, court depositions, old letters his mother wrote about him and other documents ranging from transcripts of HH's phone calls to his pilot logs. Some of the highlights of their findings as described in their report included his fear of germs which existed throughout his life. He developed intricate compulsions to protect himself from germs. For example, he wrote a staff manual on how to open a can of peaches including directions for removing the label, scrubbing the can down until it was bare metal, washing it again and pouring the contents into a bowl without touching the can to the bowl. Most important they believed his OCD often interfered with his logical, decision making which was required of him as the head of a multi-million-dollar enterprise. Also, they believed that most of what were called "eccentric" behaviors were due to OCD. The most serious result of his OCD likely accentuated by his poor hearing and TBI's, were the airplane crashes that appeared in most cases to simply be a result of some irrational pilot decisions. Some of these non-sensical decisions are described in upcoming chapters.

Historically and traditionally OCD has been considered a most disdained and misunderstood disease.[3,17] After all, a person who repeatedly does aimless behaviors like hand washing, checking door closings, or obsessing over germs is not normal. In the 17th and 18th centuries persons with OCD were generally thought to be inhabited by the devil and that God was unhappy with the individual.[3] Persecution and various forms of isolation could befall the unfortunate, afflicted individual. In the 19th century psychiatrists generally thought OCD was disordered intellect and deficient will. It was not until midway through the 20th century that OCD began to be recognized as a bonafide medical illness. Even so, many observers of HH and other persons with the disease even today consider obsessions and compulsions to be one of poor character and motivation. It was not until the late 1950's and 1960's that the post-World War II, pharmacologic development machinery really got pumping. Despite modern criticism over the costs of pharmaceuticals, the industry started to understand mental diseases such as OCD, schizophrenia, and manic depression in the 1950's and 1960's and began to develop pharmaceutical agents to control them. One of the great pharmacologic breakthroughs was the discovery of a class of drugs known as benzodiazepines. The first was chlordiazepoxide (Librium®) brought to market in 1960 and the second was diazepam (Valium®) marketed in 1963. The Physician's Desk Reference in 1965 stated the drug "is of use in dealing with anxiety reactions stemming from stressful circumstances or whenever somatic complaints are concomitants of emotional factors. It is useful in psychoneurotic states manifested by tension, fear, and fatigue." Hughes' personal physician, Dr. Norman Crane, started him on diazepam (Valium®) to assist sleep, and control his attacks of heart racing (PAT). Unexpectedly, diazepam appeared to reduce HH's germaphobia and other OCD symptoms.

OCD is now known to primarily be a dysfunction of serotonin activity in the brain. Other brain chemicals including dopamine and glutamate may also have abnormal metabolism and contribute to OCD.[9,11,45] OCD does not just spontaneously occur in normal persons. It is mainly hereditary as evidenced by his mother who clearly had OCD. Brain trauma including strokes may rarely cause the disorder. It is now an official psychiatric disease and is listed in the "Diagnostic and Statistical Manual of Mental Disorders." It is also now listed each year, beginning only about 3 years ago, in the yearly physician's handbook, "Current Therapy."[21] Whether or not it is more common today is unknown but even primary care medical practitioners recognize and diagnose OCD. "Current Therapy" provides a quick reference Table to assist primary care physicians and nurse practitioners in making a diagnosis of OCD. You will note in the table that many of HH's obsessions and compulsions are listed.

EXAMPLES OF COMMON OBSESSIONS AND COMPULSIONS	
Obsessions	**Compulsions**
Contamination or infection (germaphobia")	Avoidance of people or situations perceived as dirty, infectious, or corrupting; excessive cleaning or use of protective materials (surgical gloves, masks, sanitizer)
Control: Fear of losing control of speech or actions in public; making inappropriate comments; doing shameful or hurtful activities in public; inviting ridicule or negative reactions from others	Avoidance of others and public places; guarded behavior and curtailed speech to minimize contact with others
Religious, especially unworthiness, sinfulness, guilt	Praying, ritualizing acts of penance, seeking forgiveness (expression depends on religious belief/tradition of patient)
Sexual: concerns about acting inappropriately or being deviant	Avoidance of sexual situations, materials
Symmetry, contractures, precision	Arranging, ordering, scheduling, checking "correcting" work of others
Violence; fear of harming others or becoming dangerous	Vigilance attention to violent incidents, requiring reassurance

Adapted from Current Therapy 2020, page 797.[10]

Today there is not only understanding of the genetic biochemical abnormalities that cause OCD, but there are several therapeutic drugs and psychotherapeutic techniques that are usually effective in controlling OCD.[6,9,11,13,21] For this reason, persons with OCD are not very visible in society and do not generate the disdain and hostility that befell HH and those persons who lived with OCD prior to his time. HH was crippled by OCD throughout his life, even when he was a recluse. HH had a "germ free zone" which aides or even his physicians couldn't enter. He did not believe germs could come from him, just from the outside. If it had not been for the January 29,1928 plane crash, the medical saga of HH may not have taken such a bizarre course. As it was, however, after this day 24-year-old HH had the combined health problems of hereditary OCD, partial deafness, and TBI. Unfortunately, his uncontrolled OCD undoubtedly played a major role that led to his disastrous crash in 1928 as well as those that followed. Fortunately, the first drug to partially control OCD, diazepam (Valium®), was invented in 1963, and HH's physician started him on it shortly thereafter. Hughes took diazepam (Valium®) for the last 10 years of his life and this drug appeared to suppress, but not eliminate, some of his OCD symptoms. Unfortunately, biologic understanding and treatment for OCD was not available during the early life of HH. Had it been, HH would likely have had quite a different life and may have been able to put his mechanical and inventive genius to even greater accomplishments than the considerable ones he was able to give.

5. The Era of Traumatic Brain Injuries 1928-1951

""Cumulative Head Trauma Takes Over"

It seems impossible or implausible, but HH went on to have as many as 11 additional incidents of significant trauma after his "Hell's Angels" plane crash and coma in 1928. Several of these incidents resulted in head trauma known as a concussion, and at least four more resulted in unconsciousness and coma. Every one of these incidents may have injured his brain. At least some accentuated his OCD, as did his first TBI. Some of his traumatic events between 1928 and 1951 were so horrendous that he miraculously survived these events and maintained enough mental capacity and ability to run his various business enterprises. Much has been written about many of HH's exploitations that were either non-sensical or inappropriate. While this book makes no judgements on his business, political, or romantic activities, extremely poor judgements were clearly the cause of some of his traumatic events. Some of his abysmal decisions that led to head trauma incidents are described here.

Today we know a lot about TBI's. Studies in football players, boxers, and military veterans have determined that head injury, especially if repeated, causes a form of long-term brain dysfunction.[18,19,25,26,29] The biologic mechanism is tissue damage that produces a protein called "tau" which is deposited in brain tissue like mud in a hornet's nest.[29,37] The official scientific name is "chronic traumatic encephalopathy."[37] Usually, however, the term traumatic brain injury (TBI) is simply the moniker used in medical practice and which is used here.

Mary Lee Etsy and Carol Shifflett in their 2014 seminal book, "Conquering Concussion," were the first to report that many of the behaviors and symptoms exhibited by HH were caused by head trauma.[12] They brought their HH investigation directly to me as they correctly believed that his head trauma was an overlooked component of his life and medical saga. In their book they identified several famous persons besides Hughes, who, in retrospect, suffered TBI and exhibited bizarre and even destructive behavior. For example, in January 1536, Henry VIII was knocked unconscious and nearly died during a jousting contest. Historians believe the head trauma Henry suffered left the monarch with permanent brain damage that contributed to his increasingly erratic behavior later in life. Just four months after the accident Henry ordered the beheading of his wife, Anne Boleyn, as punishment for possibly spurious charges of infidelity. Mary Lincoln, the wife of Abraham Lincoln, had extensive education and excellent financial and organizational skills. In the early part of their marriage, she was an important power behind Abraham. Unfortunately, after a carriage accident she developed a despicable personality and became a recluse. In 1976 Elvis Presley had many health issues after falling, hitting his head, and lapsing into unconsciousness. In fact, he could hardly perform after his head trauma and he died within two years.

An analysis and cataloguing of traumatic events in the lifetime of HH is astounding. He had twelve known traumatic events and, on at least five occasions, lost consciousness. The key point to be made is that he undoubtedly suffered some permanent mental effects and other complications that compounded his OCD. For example, several medical complications including hormone deficiencies, autoimmune manifestations such as arthritis and muscle aches, headaches, and mental impairments that decrease memory, reasoning capacity, and reading ability may occur with TBI.[20,26,34,44] In other words, he inherited OCD and acquired TBI which gave him two disorders now known to cause a variety of medical and behavioral symptoms.

HOWARD HUGHES TRAUMATIC EVENTS	
YEAR	
1928	Plane crash filming "Hell's Angels." He was unconscious.
1932	Automobile accident. Hit head on windshield. Required sutures.
1935	Crash landed his H-1 racing plane in a beet field.
1936	Struck and killed a pedestrian while driving.
1940	Head-on car crash with HH's head pitched forward shattering the glass. Knocked unconscious.
1943	Sea plane crash on Lake Mead. Unconscious.
1944	Automobile accident with lacerations on face requiring sutures.
1945	Faith Domergue repeatedly smashed into HH's car with her car.
1945	Ava Gardner clobbered HH with a bronze bell and hardwood chair. HH lost consciousness.
1945	Fashion designer, Oleg Cassini, clobbered HH with a two-by-four after catching him with his wife.
1946	Crash of XF-11 experimental plane. Unconscious.
1951	Beating by ex-football player, Glen Davis, who was divorced but courting Terry Moore as was Hughes. Sustained fractures of ribs and face.

Hughes had at least four automobile accidents. He hit his head on the windshield in three. Seatbelts were not used in the first part of the last century. In one, he killed a passenger when he swerved to avoid another car. Little has been recorded about two of the auto accidents, but he hit his head in both and they required suturing of lacerations on his face or scalp.

In 1940, he was knocked unconscious after an auto accident. The concussion was so severe that he was placed in an intensive care unit. He blamed the accident on Ginger Rogers to whom he was engaged. She would not accompany him to a dentist appointment which upset him. At about the time of the accident Rogers found out that he was courting other women, so she came to his hospital room and threw her engagement ring at him which ended their relationship.

Hughes had a most serious, lucky to live, airplane crash in 1943. He had a great interest in developing planes for the military needs of World War II. He was developing an amphibian plane for the Army known as the Sikorsky S-43. It was a twin engine capable of operating off land or water. On May 17, 1943 Hughes along with an Army corps engineer named Charles W. Von Rosenberg and three other persons were to give the Sikorsky a final test run on Lake Mead in Nevada before turning the plane over to the Army. HH flew the plane and it lifted beautifully off the runway. It initially landed on the lake in what appeared to be a flawless landing in the water. Without warning the 10-ton Sikorsky began to pitch forward on its nose and veered sharply right. Before Hughes could react, the plane turned in the water and began skipping sideways. Hughes and two of the passengers survived but, two others did not. HH was dazed and suffered a concussion. After his plane crash on Lake Mead in 1943, HH clearly had mental difficulties. While convalescing he reportedly made the same request for aspirin 15 times. Dr. Vernon Mason is reported to have said, "Howard, get away from everything before you have to be committed. You're going to kill yourself." A federal investigation of the crash determined that there had been a mix-up between Hughes and the ground crew. The plane had been incorrectly loaded, altering the plane's center of gravity. The difference was apparently enough to throw the plane off balance when it touched down in the water.

The next year HH had what was called a "nervous breakdown." Exactly what his symptoms were is unknown. He did tell a government panel that he was "exhausted" and needed to take time off work. Within the next two years HH had three additional episodes of trauma which may have affected his brain. In early 1945 he was engaged to a teenage star named Faith Domergue. She caught HH with Ava Gardner while they were driving home from the Coconut Grove grand opening. Domergue saw them and HH pulled his Cadillac into a Farmer's Market parking lot. Faith backed her roadster up and repeatedly crashed her car into the passenger side door. Hughes was not hospitalized but the incident was traumatic enough to demolish both cars. Later in 1945 he was courting Ava Gardner and he had proposed marriage to her four times. He received information that Mickey Rooney was slipping in and out of Gardner's bedroom at night, so Howard secretly crept into her house and hid in her bedroom to catch any involvement between Rooney and Gardner. I have been unable to document whether he hid in the closet or under the bed, but at some point, Gardner awoke to find Hughes standing over her. After a few confronting words Hughes grabbed her by the shoulders and slapped her repeatedly. Ava groped around; found an authentic eighteenth-century bronze bell, aimed it at his head, and threw it at him. The metal sliced open Howard's head and he collapsed to the floor. Gardner grabbed a hardwood chair and hit him. HH lost consciousness and required hospitalization. He had two teeth knocked out and a splintered jaw. This incident caused Noah Dietrich and HH's physician, Dr. Vernon Mason, to believe that he had become addicted to psychodrama and danger, both real and imagined, whether it came from staring at death in an untested airplane or from confronting jealous men or women in romantic affairs.

Hughes' interests in Hollywood were films and women. He was almost completely lacking in social skills, so he relied on money and gifts to lure them into bed. If that did not work, he would propose a marriage that never seemed to happen. His behavior was manipulative and often sadistic. He had his women of interest (and any potential rivals) followed and spied on, from who they were seeing, to the contents of their medical records. Sometimes the women, their husbands or lovers struck back.

In 1945, HH was dating an alluring star named Gene Tierney. She married an upscale fashion designer named Oleg Cassini who confronted Hughes at one of Jack Benny's dinner parties and told him to stay away from his wife. Later, however, Tierney and Hughes snuck off to Las Vegas. When they returned Cassini caught them and clobbered Hughes with a two-by-four.

In 1946 HH crashed his experimental XF-11 reconnaissance plane and miraculously survived. Details of the crash and his medical care are in later chapters. This flight was a first-time experimental flight for this aircraft and Hughes made such unbelievable bad decisions in flying the plane that he must have been impaired by his OCD and prior TBI's. He grossly ignored the test protocol which strictly limited:

- Fuel to 600 gallons
- Landing gear down at all times
- Flight time of 45 minutes

Testing was to have been done at the Army Test Flight Base in the barren Mojave Desert. Instead, Hughes persuaded the Air Force to let him test the plane at his Culver City headquarters. At flight time he violated the test protocol by the following actions:

- Loaded 1,200 gallons of fuel. He apparently planned to fly further despite a known oil leak.
- Raised the landing gear (which may have jammed).
- Flew for 75 minutes.

At 30 minutes beyond the prescribed flight duration time, the propellers malfunctioned due to an oil leak which was noticed several times during the test. No wonder the plane crashed into heavily populated Beverly Hills.

The last known trauma to HH occurred in 1951. In 1949 he apparently married Terry Moore, an actress, while on a boat cruise. There is no legal marriage license attesting to this marriage, and he and Moore broke up later. She later married and divorced Glen Davis, a former West Point and Los Angeles Rams football star. Using his usual poor judgement when it came to women, HH sent Terry's engagement ring to Davis. He was enraged and subsequently attacked HH rebreaking some of his ribs and chin. Hughes probably suffered another episode of TBI in this beating. Exactly where and how this beating occurred has been a matter of debate and conjecture. Donald Bartlett and James Steele, the celebrated, award-winning journalists who wrote "Howard Hughes: His Life and Madness" state that Terry was at her mother's house in Los Angeles and both Hughes and Davis showed up at the same time. Hughes tried to shake his hand in a reconciliation and sporting gesture, but Davis slapped the outstretched hand and proceeded to attack Hughes. Terry Moore's mother threw herself on top of Hughes to prevent bodily harm. Regardless of the precise facts about the Davis assault, it is likely that the 1951 trauma at the hands of Davis accelerated and worsened his combined impairments of OCD and TBI.

Esty and Shifflett, after studying all available reports, were able to determine that HH's most obvious symptoms of TBI and OCD began shortly after his 1928 "Hell's Angels" plane crash. He started exhibiting these symptoms and behaviors:

- Germ phobia and compulsions such as sorting and counting the peas on his plate (there had to be 12 and all had to be the same size).
- Poor self-awareness, self-care, and grooming.

- Extreme paranoia and controlling behavior, including an entire staff of spies and wire tappers to follow his women, rivals, and competitors.
- Extreme and indiscreet sexual behavior.

After the 1928 crash, the man with the superb memory began repeating himself, having forgotten that he had given the same order seconds before. One day, business manager Noah Dietrich logged over 30 repetitions of the same sentence on a note pad.

He became famous for working non-stop for two to three days at a time. Whether this was single-minded dedication to work or simple inability to sleep, the certain result was sleep deprivation. The stress and strain of managing multiple projects was enormous, and his symptoms and behaviors were made worse by the workload and responsibility.

Hughes suffered from two nervous breakdowns. The term "nervous breakdown" is not an actual medical term. It is not a diagnosis. It does not describe a specific mental illness. It was a general term commonly used in the 1940's and 50's and indicated an inability to function normally in daily life due to overwhelming physical or emotional stress, depression, anxiety, and/or exhaustion. In 1944 he took about seven months off to recover from a "nervous breakdown." He apparently had another episode called a "nervous breakdown" in 1957. His specific symptoms and any medical treatments given are unknown.

After the 1946 airplane crash, he began to exhibit even more bizarre behaviors. For example, in 1947, he reportedly locked himself inside a dark screening room for four months. He sat naked and alone, living only on milk, chocolate bars, and pecans, watching movies over and over. Not understood at the time,

Photophobia (light sensitivity) is a symptom of both TBI and severe, chronic pain.

After this incident he started to periodically withdraw from public life and become a recluse. After the mid-1950's he was rarely seen. He continued to run his business affairs from his dark room with a steady stream of memos scrawled on yellow legal pads. These sometimes included absurdly detailed instructions such as a nine-step essay on the correct procedures for opening and removing fruit from a can.

There are no reports that he was drinking alcohol and was inebriated as a cause of his crashes. We now know that a person with OCD, TBI, and hearing deficit would be a hazard behind the wheel of a car or plane. HH essentially gave up driving in the early 1950's. It is unknown whether he had a driver's license. By 1950 he required regular dosages of codeine for his pain, so it is highly likely that his doctors advised him against driving. HH had regular chauffeurs, starting in the early 1950's, and there are no reports of auto accidents or other traumatic events after 1951. HH, himself, may have realized that his medical disorders would impair driving or flying.

TBI is now considered a serious medical issue and physicians treat it as a disease. About 1.7 million Americans suffer a TBI each year. A variety of medical, physical, and psychiatric measures are currently being used in therapy for TBI. These include electromagnetic therapies, psychological relearning techniques, biochemical surrogates, and hormone restoration. Prevention for athletes and workers who are at risk for TBI is a modern-day concern. For example, special head gear is now a requirement in several sports. Listed here is a table of the primary symptoms of TBI – HH had many of them. If TBI causes pain it is medically called "central pain syndrome." Other than occasional headaches, HH did not exhibit chronic pain until after his 1946 plane crash. A variety of drugs for mental illness and disorders are now usually attempted in patients with TBI in hopes of getting a reduction in symptoms. HH was given diazepam (Valium®) during the last ten years of his life, and this drug may have reduced some TBI symptoms. After he started diazepam (Valium®) there are no reports of dastardly business decisions or reprehensible public actions. In fact, he essentially reinvented Las Vegas after he started the drug.

In summary, by the time HH was 25 years old he had hereditary OCD, partial deafness, and TBI's. It is no wonder that he went on to have about a dozen traumatic events and became notorious for some of his public offensive behaviors. Not until late in the last century were OCD or TBI even considered medical disorders. Until the last few years of his life there were no drugs to attempt treatment. Today, it is different. Both conditions are recognized as serious medical problems. Both are now listed in medical textbooks with treatment suggestions for doctors to use. We can only speculate what fate would have befallen HH if either one or both conditions had been recognized early in his life and treated with today's medical measures.

COMMON SYMPTOMS AFTER TRAUMATIC BRAIN INURY (TBI)
Cognition
Memory problems, especially short-term
Preservation (repeated requests of demands)
Slowed thoughts, difficulty finding words
Decreased focus/concentration
Problems with organization, sequencing, and decision-making
Spatial disorientation, loss of sense of direction
Loss of familiar skills
Physical and Sensory
Headache, nausea, and body pain
Visual problems: light sensitivity, gritty eyes, difficulty reading
Severe fatigue and apathy
Physical weakness
Gastro-intestinal problems, especially constipation
Sensory dysfunction including abnormal cold and sweating
Hallucinations: auditory, visual, olfactory, or tactile
Changes in food preferences
Slowed reaction time and poor balance
Altered speech
Sleep disruptions from insomnia to inability to stay awake
Movement disorders and muscle spasms
Seizures, from "blanking out" to grand mall
Tear ducts that squirt fluid (on blowing nose)
Emotional
Loss of a complex (or adult) sense of humor
Emotional lability/ "roller-coaster" emotions

Impulsiveness and risky behavior
Anger, explosiveness, rage, despair
Flat affect
Loss of social skills
Obsessive talking or writing
Poor hygiene and grooming
Depression, apathy, and detachment
Anxiety and panic attacks
Paranoia
Many of the above symptoms characterize Howard Hughes. The recognition, identification, and cataloguing of these symptoms were developed since 2000 and were not even considered to be associated with head trauma during the life of HH.
Adapted from Conquering Concussion.[12]

6. The Beginning of the End – 1946

""Miracle of Survival""

Among all HH's traumatic events, an airplane crash in 1946 was the one that changed his life and health the most. What is more, at the time of HH's death in 1976, no one initially considered that his plane crash in 1946 was the cause of his death, or that the plane crash was undoubtedly related to his OCD and TBI. After all, an interval of 30 years had interceded, and it seemed incongruous that kidney failure could be tied to such a long-ago event. The connection between his plane crash and cause of death became clear at his autopsy. Post-mortem toxicology analysis pinpointed the relationship between the plane crash and kidney failure. My 1978 report to the government, which is in the appendix of this book, describes the connection in detail. The tie between kidney failure and the plane crash is that Dr. Vern Mason, his personal physician, initiated pain treatment after his crash with a codeine compound that contained a kidney-toxic drug called phenacetin. In 1946 no one realized that long term use of this drug could cause kidney failure. Phenacetin was a very popular over the counter (OTC), pain reliever until it was pulled from the commercial market after HH's death. Naturally, his demise called dramatic attention to phenacetin's potential complications. In much of the last century, phenacetin was a component of the ubiquitous, pain reliever known simply as "APC." This compound was aspirin, phenacetin, and caffeine. The three components were sold as one treatment agent as well as combined with codeine.

The previous chapter describes the poor judgement HH used in violating the ground rules for flying the XF-11 experimental plane. Surviving the crash was a medical miracle. In their excellent book, "The Untold Story: Howard Hughes," Peter Brown and Pat Broeske provide a detailed account of the miracle, and their description is the basis of the report given here. Also included here is information that I personally obtained from Dr. Lawrence Chaffin, the surgeon who saved HH's life after the crash.

On July 7, 1946 HH took off from his private airport in Culver City to flight test the US Army reconnaissance plane, the XF-11. Within two hours the plane failed and crashed in Beverly Hills after hitting three houses. The plane split into pieces. A marine sergeant by the name of William Lloyd Durbin saw the fiery crash and with the help of an unidentified fireman who was a passerby pulled HH out of the wreckage. Medics initially transported HH by ambulance to the Beverly Hills Emergency Hospital. The emergency physician recognized that HH's lungs were filling with fluid, so they put him in an oxygen tent and immediately sent him to Good Samaritan Hospital that had a burn unit. By the time he reached Good Samaritan, he was losing so much blood that transfusions were started. His lungs were filled with fluid. When HH reached Good Samaritan, he informed their staff doctors that he would wait for his own doctors – Drs. Vern Mason and Lawrence Chaffin. They both arrived within two hours after the crash and went immediately to work on HH. Their long clinical experience including military medical service literally saved HH. Within about 30 minutes Dr. Mason had drained 3400 cc of bloody fluid from Hughes chest cavity and started another transfusion. At one-point HH asked Dr. Mason, "How am I doing?", Dr. Mason replied, "I am not going to lie to you, Howard. You may not live." "Do what you can" he mumbled, "I'm prepared." Mason and Chaffin worked steadily on Hughes for about eight hours into the next day after the crash. At one point he fell into shock and a coma. Within about 36 hours Hughes required constant transfusions and his lungs had to be drained twice. By dawn on July 10, about 48 hours after the crash, his blood pressure returned to normal, and his crushed left lung started to function.

With this upturn in cardiopulmonary function Dr. Verne Mason gave his first press conference in the lobby of Good Samaritan. He exclaimed, "My patient is truly a Man of Steel, and he is crawling back to health from injuries that would have killed most men. He is not out of danger yet, but he has a terrific will to live. That alone might save him." Then Dr. Mason provided the ultimate photo opportunity. He held up Hughes partly charred, "worse-for-wear" lucky fedora hat which had been recovered from the wreckage.

By the fourth day (July 11), Hughes was able to sit up and eat one graham cracker. By nightfall, however, his left lung again filled with fluid, and his blood pressure dropped again causing him to lose consciousness. Howard asked Dr. Mason, "Am I going to live?" Dr. Mason looked him in the eye and replied, "I don't know Howard. I sure can't guarantee it."

On July 12, the 5th day, he again hovered near death and his chest again filled for the 3rd time requiring drainage. Amazing, on the next day he had remarkable improvement with lung function that continued to improve with the necessity of only one drainage. He was taken off oxygen for the first time since the crash.

Hughes remained in the hospital between July 7 and August 11, or about five weeks. While in the hospital he started doing business in the last two weeks of his stay. The first thing he did was have telephones installed and turned up the volume to accommodate the hearing defect that he had since his teenage years.

The doctors who saved HH were the last of a breed of physicians that are now quite rare. Both had military trauma experience and knew how to balance transfusions, lung drainage, and oxygen administration, while providing pain relief with morphine. Make one mistake and the game is over. HH had one characteristic that seemed to bail him out of his poor judgements and decisions. He hired the best people and paid them well. Noah Dietrich, for example, was an excellent pick to run HH's early empire. The life-saving medical care he received after the crash also showed this characteristic. He had hired Drs. Mason and Chaffin who were among the absolute best physicians that LA had to offer in those years.

The doctor closest to HH was Vern Mason, MD. He became his personal physician just after Howard moved to LA in the late 1920's. He remained his primary physician for about 35-40 years until about 1960. HH selected Dr. Mason in 1953 to head the scientific advisory board for the Howard Hughes Medical Institute. Dr. Mason moved to Miami around 1960 and died in 1965. The move was to the supervise the research sponsored by the Institute since it was headquartered there.

Verne Mason was born in Wapello, Iowa in 1889. He received his MD degree from John Hopkins University in 1915. As an internal medicine resident at John Hopkins in 1922, he studied and named sickle cell disease. He established his medical practice in LA after residency and became the internist to many Hollywood personalities and reportedly diagnosed the cause and treated General of the Army John J. Pershing who had lapsed suddenly into a coma. He served as a highly decorated medical officer in both World Wars. This experience undoubtedly helped him save the life of HH after his 1946 plane crash since he sustained the type of injuries seldom seen outside of military combat.

Dr. Lawrence Chaffin was also superbly qualified and had earned elite respect in the LA medical community. He was born on June 1, 1892 and received his medical license in 1917. He attended Harvard Medical School and Residency and began his surgical practice in LA in 1922. At age 68 he achieved Emeritus status at the University of California. At the time of HH's death in 1976, Dr. Chaffin was 84 years of age and still practicing.

Dr. Mason called Dr. Chaffin to assist him in the care of HH in 1932 after Hughes suffered lacerations from an auto accident. Dr. Chaffin intermittently cared for HH between 1932 and the day he died in 1976. His chore was to deal with surgical matters which were primarily injuries such as lacerations and concussions in HH's early life. He took care of HH's rectal prolapse, needle injection complications, and pressure sores in the last three years of his life.

Dr. Chaffin, under oath in the trial of United States versus Thain, in 1978, gave a specific account to the jury about the injuries suffered in HH's 1946 plane crash. His verbatim description of HH's injuries is given here as they form the basis of most of HH's later life of secrecy and medical care. This account amply highlights the miracle of survival following his crash and the necessity of opioids and other drugs for the rest of his life. The severity of his injuries is now known to cause nervous system alterations which may lead to a relatively rare condition called "Intractable Pain Syndrome" (IPS). Simply stated, injuries of the severity that befell HH are not cured or resolved and forever change the victim's life.

For historic preservation, Dr. Chaffin's "Verbatim Account of HH'S Injuries in His 1946 Airplane Crash" is given here:

Beginning with the skin. He had multiple burns involving his left ear, his left chest, his left abdominal wall, the little finger side of his left hand, and his left buttocks.

Now, in small spotted areas there were third degree burns, meaning that they went through the skin and left permanent scars. For example, he had a scar on his left little finger that kept it from extending fully. It was pulled down a little.

He had an injury involving his fifth and sixth cervical vertebrae, those being the two vertebrae at the base of the neck.

The lateral articular facets-those are the joints on the side which join the sixth to the seventh vertebrae, there was a fracture extending through them. And in a lateral x-ray view of the neck, he had a very slight forward displacement of the body of the 6th cervical vertebrae on the body of the 7th.

He had fractures of the first, 2nd, 3rd, and I believe the 4th right ribs, with a separation of the 1st costochondral junction. That means the joint on the side of the breastbone to which the first rib joins the sternum.

He had fractures of the 1,2,3,4,5,6,7,8,9 left ribs with a fracture of the left clavicle.

He had extensive subcutaneous emphysema. That means that he had air under the skin. If you felt the skin, you could feel it crepitate, air bubbles under the skin, meaning that he had a puncture of a lung in connection with his rib fractures.

He had a large hemorrhage into his left chest cavity, the cavity where the left lung is. This pushed his heart over to the right so that the heart was beyond the midline. Normally the heart is over the left side of the chest. We thought, also, that he had a contusion of his heart wall. We thought that because he had a very rapid pulse for a few days.

He also had a hemorrhage into his mediastinum. Now the mediastinum is the space immediately behind the breastbone through which passed the esophagus, which is the tube between your mouth and your stomach, and the trachea or windpipe. He had enough pressure in that area so that he could not swallow for about four days.

He had multiple bruises and abrasions from being jostled about.

The above list of injuries sustained in the crash clearly shows that HH was not only lucky to survive, but the severity of the injuries was destined to require opioids for pain relief and intensive medical care for the remainder of his life that totaled about 30 years.

After the crash HH grew a mustache to cover some of his facial scarring that resulted from the crash. As far as is known, he continually kept his mustache until his death in 1976. Regrettably, I have been unable to find any statement by HH about his personal inner-feelings, goals or visions after his lifesaving stay at Good Samaritan Hospital. He clearly knew that death had been close at hand and that he was lucky to walk out of the hospital. Persons who have had near-death experiences have been a significant part of my medical career. They all change their life in some way and are grateful. They all thank their God and guiding Spirits. All make some vows and know they have a debt to repay. Some are eager to talk about it. Others, like HH, may never talk about it or only relate their new life plan to their doctor. HH certainly contributed a great deal to society after his crash, but his visions or desires were never publicly voiced. By his actions, however, he went right back to work after the crash and even successfully piloted the second XF-11 plane about a year after his crash. Unfortunately, the injuries and burns he sustained in the crash were not going to let him escape unscathed and simply return to the health and life he had before the crash.

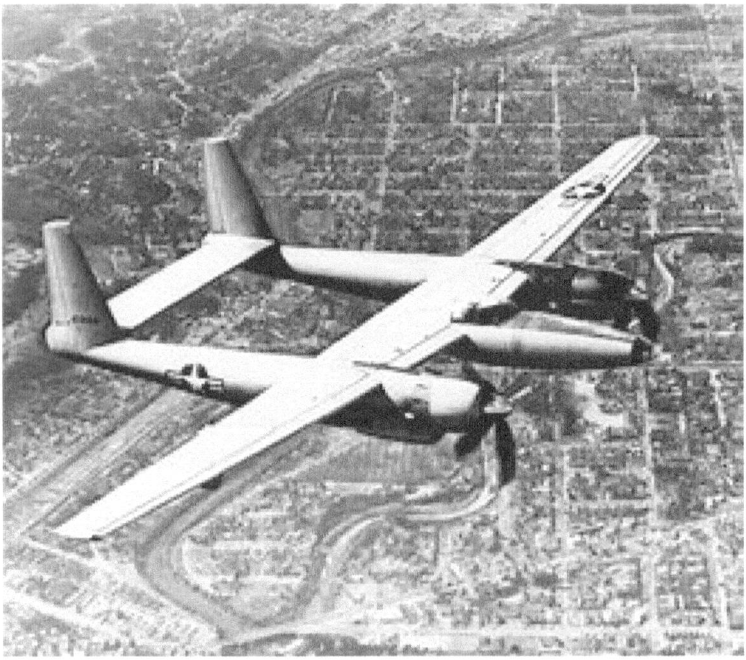

The XF-11 experimental plane in which Hughes crashed -1946

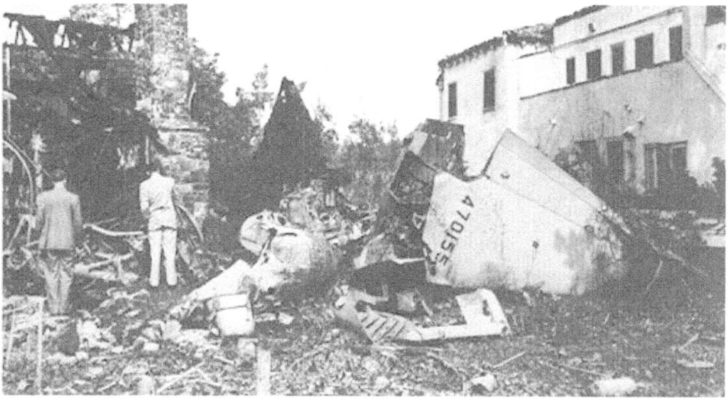

This is the scene of the XF-11 crash. Hughes miraculously survived but was left with multiple injuries, impairments, and the intractable pain syndrome.

7. Survival and Change of Life: 1946-1961

""Health Deteriorates and Reclusiveness Sets In""

Miraculously, HH survived his 1946 plane crash. He clearly had a near death experience. To survive the type of burns and injuries that HH sustained in the crash, three things must go right. First, one must have a real "will to live." Second, you better have some good doctors, and third, you will in some ways have to change your life. You cannot go back. HH lived 30 years after his near-death crash, and there is ample evidence that he did all three of the things that one has to do to survive such an ordeal.

Just after Hughes entered the hospital after the crash, he was prescribed morphine for pain by Drs. Mason and Chaffin. He continued periodic morphine until he was discharged. As an outpatient, he continued under the care of Dr. Mason who started HH on oral codeine compound upon discharge from the hospital. This was a drug formulation that contained aspirin, caffeine, and phenacetin. Shortly after his hospital discharge Dr. Mason stated to the media that HH was still in pain due to his injuries and that codeine was necessary. No other public notice or information was ever again given about the medical care that HH received over the next 30 years until his death. Medical records or typical doctors' notes normally kept in a practitioner's office were apparently not kept or were never made available to the public and disappeared.

After his 34 day stay at Good Samaritan Hospital, he initially moved into Cary Grant's rented villa to recuperate. Later he moved from one hotel to another and one house to another throughout recovery, although it is unknown how long his "recovery" lasted. His actions after the crash seemed to imply that he wanted to return to aviation and redeem himself. For example, within a year he had recovered enough to successfully test fly the second FX-11.

His business and political activities in the late 1940's and early 1950's are legend and somewhat of a testament to his recovery and enhanced motivation. In 1947 he flew the Hercules Giant Plane popularly known as the "Spruce Goose." He also, in 1947, appeared before the Senate War Investigating Committee and was very articulate and persuasive. In 1948 he acquired RKO Production Company and formed Hughes Helicopters. He restarted his womanizing shortly after his crash as his sexual abilities were surprisingly left intact. HH began to withdraw from public appearances shortly after the Glen Davis physical beating in 1951. On January 12, 1957 he married Jean Peters. The marriage lasted 13 years until they divorced in 1971, at which time she claimed she had not seen him for several years having separated in the early 1960's. Within about 10 years, however, he would, like other persons with IPS, become impotent.

During the first 15 years after his 1946 air crash, the only medication that HH is known to have taken on a regular basis is oral codeine compound. There are no reports or indications that the drug ever made him drowsy or sedated. Interestingly, writings about HH seem to report fewer OCD symptoms such as irrational fear of germs and repetitive actions. It is entirely plausible and possible that codeine compound controlled some of his OCD and TBI symptoms. It is known, however, that significant deterioration of his physical health began in the mid-1950's about six to eight years after the crash. At some point in his recovery HH decided to give up film making, test piloting planes, and even driving a car. His activities were clearly directed at investing his money, acquiring businesses, and building his empire. HH also appeared to function relatively well physically and mentally for about the first 10 years after his crash. Between 1955 and 1960 his physical body began to show some of the long-term sequelae of damage to joints, nerves, and muscles. He seldom walked after 1960 and his neck became permanently fixated in a bent position so that he had to sleep in a partial sitting position. He required a "two pillow-pillow." This was a hard pillow in a pillowcase next to his back and a regular pillow was on top to be placed against his head and neck.

Interestingly, HH moved forward in 1953 with a long-held wish and vision to form the Howard Hughes Medical Institute. Formation of the Institute was done by donating all of Hughes Aircraft stock that handsomely endowed the Institute. While some critics claim this creation was merely a tax dodge and business deal, the timing suggests that HH may have known that deterioration was settling in and he needed to follow through with a lifetime dream.

Dr. Vernon Mason remained the personal physician to HH and prescribed codeine and any other needed drugs to HH between the crash in 1946 and his retirement in 1961. Dr. Norman Crane, an office associate of Dr. Mason, assisted in the care of HH starting in 1955. Dr. Crane took over HH's care and the prescribing of drugs in 1961. Other than codeine it is unknown if Dr. Mason or Dr. Crane regularly prescribed any additional drugs.

Interestingly, the Federal Government obtained a document written by HH on October 2, 1958. It is called "Operating Memorandum" with the subject being, "Instruction from HRH Regarding Securing and Processing Prescriptions." This memorandum is published verbatim in the appendix. It confirms that HH was married to Jean Peters and living in one or more LA hotels. It is also clear that he was getting codeine. No names of physicians or drugs, however, are stated in the memorandum. Most important it clearly states that neither his nor Jean Peters real names are to be used on prescriptions. This is, of course, illegal. Dr. Crane who shared office space with Dr. Mason, and was, in effect his partner, supplied HH with 36 codeine prescriptions between 1955 and 1961.

Just how much physiologic deterioration set in during the first 15 years after his 1946 crash is imprecisely known, but some degree occurred as would be expected considering his injuries, burns, and pain. His ability to ambulate began to progressively decrease in the 1950's. He discontinued his notorious affairs with women in the mid-1950's. He and Jean Peters separated around 1960. His mind, however, had to be in relatively good shape as he continued to run his empire and make financial decisions that proved to be profitable. Constant pain had set in. The worst emanated from his neck although he had some headaches, dental pain, and his skin was sometimes too sensitive to touch. By 1960, at age 55, he was saddled with OCD, TBI, partial deafness, and now he had constant pain requiring daily opioid medication. He also had a changed appearance. He wore a moustache to cover some of his facial scars, but he also had some other scars on his face and scalp. All these issues fostered an increasing reclusiveness and secret existence. Despite all his diseases, impairments, and handicaps, however, he clearly had to have a great will to live. Most people would probably "give up" if they had all his maladies.

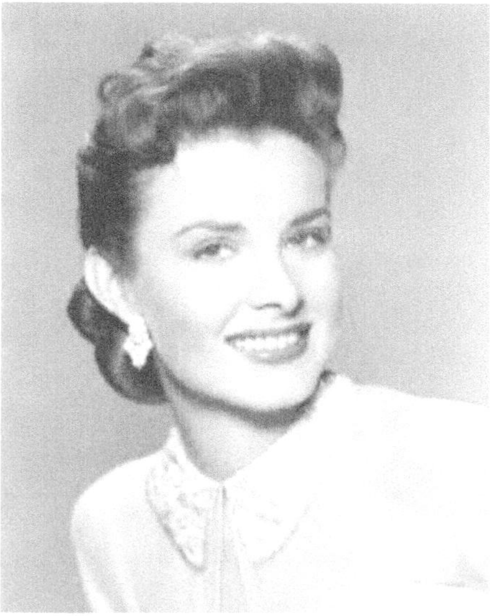

Howard married Jean Peters in 1957. They divorced in 1970. He stated to his physicians near the end of his life that she was his one true love. She is believed to have anonymously sent a bouquet of roses to his burial service and later decorated his grave.

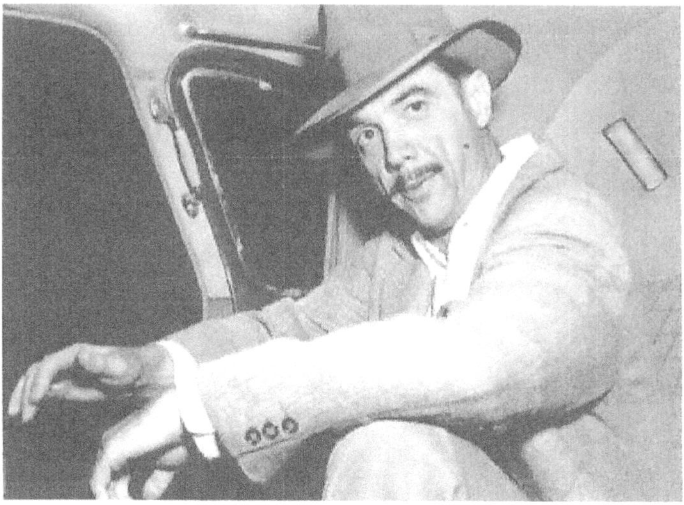

After his 1964 XF-11 crash, Hughes grew a moustache to cover scars. He always wore his lucky Fedora hat when testing an airplane.

8. Intractable Pain Syndrome Sets In: 1955-1960

""Coping with Daily Pain"

On leaving Good Samaritan Hospital in 1946, Dr. Vern Mason initiated oral codeine compound for HH as he was in pain. In the hospital he received morphine. Codeine was a natural step as it converts to morphine when it reaches the blood stream after being orally digested or injected. It was the most popular opioid pain reliever in 1946. The severity of his pain and the frequency which he needed codeine in the years immediately following his crash is not precisely known but it progressively increased. What is clear is that he had chronic, intermittent pain for about a decade after his 1946 crash. He showed minimal physiologic impairments in the 8 to 10 years after his crash. At some point after his 1946 air crash, he developed what is now called "Intractable Pain Syndrome." Circumstantial evidence suggests that this syndrome developed in his mid-50's. As described in previous chapters Glen Davis, a former football player, encountered HH in 1951 and gave him a severe physical beating. This trauma may have accelerated his switch from simple chronic pain state to IPS.

IPS is defined as "constant incurable pain with cardiovascular and endocrine (hormone) complications."[14,16,32,33,36,39,40] The switch from simple chronic pain to IPS develops when nerve damage due to an injury or disease creates and sends excess electricity into the brain and spinal cord (central nervous system, CNS). Over an extended time, this causes inflammation which destroys tissues in the CNS that normally control and limit pain.[1,25,30,42] This is a tragic development, because it is biochemicals such as endorphin, dopamine, and serotonin which are produced in healthy brain tissue that normally control and limit pain.[23,27] If enough brain tissue and biochemical production are damaged by inflammation, pain is not shut down and it becomes constant.[24,28,31]

When pain becomes constant, the cardiovascular and endocrine systems overact and produce many complications of which several were evident in HH.[16,32,36,40,41] Constant pain stimulates the pituitary and adrenal glands to produce extra amounts of the hormones, insulin, cortisol, and adrenaline.[40] Adrenaline raises blood pressure and pulse rate and may initiate cardiac arrhythmias, constriction of a coronary artery (angina), or heart attack. HH developed multiple cardiovascular complications from his IPS. He frequently had episodes of severe tachycardia with a pulse or heart rate as high as 200 beats per minute. Apparently, he started these heart racing episodes of "paroxysmal atrial tachycardia" (PAT) after his 1928 "Hell's Angels" plane crash and TBI. They became quite frequent, however, after he developed IPS. Episodes of tachycardia are often triggered by pain flares. Although HH in his reclusive years resisted most medical care including physical examinations, he became somewhat frightened by the PAT attacks. He allowed his physicians to keep an electrocardiogram machine in his hotel suite and apply pressure to his carotid arteries to stop the attack. His doctors were all aware of these episodes and had briefed each other that carotid pressure would always break the episode. HH's autopsy showed that "mild to moderate coronary arteriosclerosis was present with a single focus of 60% luminal narrowing in the mid portion of the left anterior descending artery." (See autopsy report Appendix.) In addition, the autopsy found that the "abdominal aorta distal to the renal vessels shows four ulcerated plaques with attached fibrinous thrombi." A reasonable interpretation of these findings is that HH at the time of death from renal disease was also at considerable risk to die of a heart attack or stroke in the relatively near future. One of the fibrinous thrombi could come loose and travel to the brain producing a fatal stroke. IPS causes cortisol and insulin to raise, so persons with IPS all develop a pre-diabetic or active diabetic state with cholesterol and plaque formations in arteries including the coronary arteries.

The main trauma and burn sites that caused HH to develop IPS were to his neck and chest. He initially damaged vertebrae in his neck as well as adjacent nerves and connective tissues. Over time his intervertebral discs deteriorated and collapsed onto the nerves that come out of the cervical spinal cord. This development caused severe pain which undoubtedly required even more pain control medication.

HH also suffered a complication that usually disables, demoralizes, and depresses persons with IPS – loss of bone and dental mass. The "24/7," constant pain of IPS raises cortisol and depresses production of testosterone, estradiol, progesterone, and a hormone called dehydroepiandrosterone (DHEA).[36,40,41] Cortisol elevations over time cause so much bone and dental mass to be lost that persons with IPS often feel like they are "falling apart" which is an accurate, literal feeling. HH's teeth became so deteriorated that he had a most unpleasant breath. All his doctors pleaded with him to accept dental care, but he always refused. He would not let his aides brush his teeth. This is somewhat understandable due to pain hypersensitivity which is part of IPS.[23,24,31] Loss of bone mass is called osteoporosis, and he had bone loss throughout his body. His neck was very affected. He had collapsed vertebrae due to osteoporosis and his head and neck became fixed in a forward position. By age 55 he began to have limited mobility since his hip, leg, and ankle bones had developed osteoporosis and weakness. In 1973, at age 67, he fell and fractured a hip which is common in persons with IPS. His overall height shrank from about 6'4" to about 6'0" due to osteoporosis and bone collapse.

Testosterone is a hormone that produces sex drive and the physiologic changes in a male that permits one to consummate the sex act.[44] It is also essential for bone and dental growth and repair. Much has been written about HH's sexual escapades and womanizing. It appears that he was able to carry on sexually for about 10 years after his 1946 plane crash. IPS, however, is a progressive disease fostered by inflammation in the brain and spinal cord.[2,5,14] Hormone exhaustion occurs, so persons with IPS almost always lose their sexual ability. The codeine and diazepam (Valium®) that HH required for pain control may also suppress testosterone production.[40] He married Jean Peters in 1957 but they lived in separate quarters and apart after about 1958 or 59 and they divorced in 1971. Michael Drosnin in his excellent investigative book, "Citizen Hughes" describes a pathetic event that appears to pinpoint the approximate time that IPS took its toll on HH's gonads and testosterone. In 1958 he was keeping a 16-year-old teenage beauty queen in a hideaway located in Coldwater Canyon north of Hollywood. Hughes brought her to his bungalow once to celebrate his 53rd birthday on Christmas Eve 1958. He did not see her again. She called HH a few months later and gave Howard this message overheard by her guards, "You dirty old son of a bitch. You never come to see me. I'll bet you can't even get it up anymore, you impotent old slob."

Beside HH's obvious cardiovascular and endocrine complications he had another complication of IPS that modern pain doctors like to call "central sensitization."[24,31] This means that IPS has made the nervous system oversensitive to "external stimuli." In simple terms it means that smell, light, taste, hearing, feel, or touch (See Table of Characteristics) may cause pain or discomfort. Common manifestations include light sensitivity. Persons with IPS often need to live in darkened quarters and wear sunglasses. Light causes too much pain. Some smells or noises may cause great agitation or a pain flare. It may hurt too much to brush teeth, comb hair, or cut finger and toenails. Hygiene chores may be skipped.

Even clothes touching the skin may be painful. Reports by HH aides claim that he did occasionally have his hair, beard, and nails trimmed. This probably occurred at times when his pain was stable and not in a flare. HH's teeth became so fragile and painful he had to have soft food and did not eat any solid foods, at least in the latter years of his life. Hughes' last head physician, Dr. Wilbur Thain, related that HH complained that sometimes it hurt too much to be touched and examined. Since the days of HH, names have been medically applied to the hypersensitive conditions that befell HH. Too much pain to the touch is called allodynia. The medical name attached to nerves which have been damaged by injuries such as Hughes is "Reflex Sympathetic Dystrophy" or "Chronic Regional Pain Syndrome."

Persons with IPS tend to become socially isolated and reclusive. Seen here are Tables from one of the author's studies. One Table shows the difference between those persons who have simple chronic pain of the type you typically get with such common conditions as old age arthritis, bunions, carpal tunnel, and temporomandibular joint inflammation (TMJ) and those with IPS.[14,39] The other shows characteristics of a group of 40 patients with IPS like HH. A review of the Table reveals that many of HH's symptoms and characteristics are typical of other persons with the relatively rare condition of IPS. For example, most persons with IPS shun crowds, desire isolation, and have poor balance. HH fell several times and, in 1973, fractured his hip from a fall while staying in London.

It is important to point out that the typical symptoms of OCD including germaphobia and non-sensical behaviors such as repetitive handwashing are not observed in persons who only have IPS. Also, persons with IPS are not observed to make terrible, illogical decisions or severe memory lapses which are commonly observed in persons with TBI. Unfortunately, HH had all three of these conditions, so he had multiple, seemingly unexplained symptoms and behaviors during his lifetime. What is more, the three conditions probably accentuated each other to produce the strange medical saga of HH.

CHARACTERISTICS OF SIMPLE CHRONIC AND INTRACTABLE PAIN SYNDROME	IPS	CP
Pain is Constant (24/7)	Yes	No
Treatment is Daily (Around the Clock)	Yes	No
Elevated Blood Pressure and Pulse Rate	Yes	Seldom
Elevated Temperature and Breathing Rate	Yes	No
Anorexia/Malnutrition	Yes	No
Insomnia	Yes	No
Depression, Hopelessness	Yes	No
Endocrine Abnormalities	Yes	No
Elevated Inflammatory Markers	Often	Seldom
Restriction of certain life activities (e.g., mobility)	Yes	Sometimes
Decreased capability for Requirements of Daily Living	Yes	No

CLINICAL PROFILE OF 40 PERSONS WITH THE INTRACTABLE PAIN SYNDROME			
	Symptom	**No.**	**%**
1	Constant pain – always present (24/7)	40	100
2	Pain wakes you up	39	97.5
3	Too fatigued to leave home or do normal activities	39	97.5
4	Difficulty with cognitive tasks such as memory, concentration, or letter composition	39	97.5
5	Prevents falling asleep even if fatigued or tired	38	95.0
6	Feel tired after full night's sleep	38	95.0
7	Difficulty paying attention to conversation	37	92.5
8	Fatigue and difficulty concentrating makes it difficult to interact with others	37	92.5
9	Pain moves from one body location to another	36	90.0
10	Experience extreme chronic fatigue	36	90.0
11	Difficulty finding works when speaking	36	90.0
12	Hypersensitivity to noise, lights, traffic, crowds	36	90.0
13	Experience chronic "all-over" pain	36	90.0
14	Problems with balance and falling	35	87.5
15	Blood pressure elevated much of the time	35	87.5
16	Craves sugars and starches even when full	34	85.0
17	Experience episodes of heat, sweating, and elevated temperature	33	82.5

18	Bothered by pressure of clothing or seat belt	32	80.0
19	Hands and feet are cold much of the time	32	80.0
20	Sometimes hurts to be touched	32	80.0
21	Often want to be left alone	32	80.0
22	Sensitive to touch sometimes prevents lying in bed or sitting	31	77.5
23	Pulse rate is elevated even when lying down	30	75.0
24	Lost most of appetite	29	72.5
25	Has periodic, incapacitating muscle spasms	29	72.5
26	Has a feeling of "heavy legs" making it hard to walk	29	70.0
27	Severe dental problems such as abscessed teeth	27	67.5
28	Sometimes painful to comb hair, brush teeth, or cut your nails	24	60.0

Shown here is a Table from 40 persons with IPS who are in the author's research studies. It is remarkable that the clinical symptoms and complications of these relatively rare individuals are so like each other and how well they resemble HH.

The symptomatic treatment given to HH for IPS was horrendous by today's standards, and it is not surprising that one of his treatment agents, phenacetin, led to his death. All his physicians could do, however, was prescribe what was available to them: codeine and diazepam (Valium®). There was no understanding in Hughes' day of such biologic concepts as pain causing inflammation and damage to CNS tissues. Brain chemicals such as endorphins had not been discovered. There was no knowledge that constant, severe pain can cause cardiovascular and endocrine complications. His doctors over a 30-year period prescribed codeine compound which contained aspirin, caffeine, and phenacetin, and prescribed the drug diazepam (Valium®) for about the last 10 years of his life. Clearly these two agents did not satisfactorily control his pain or adequately slow his deterioration. For example, his teeth continued to deteriorate, and his bones continued to collapse indicating that his medical treatment with codeine and diazepam did not completely control excess cortisol production. He also continued to have periodic episodes of PAT.

His treatment also had other complications besides phenacetin kidney toxicity. He had severe constipation and rectal prolapse. Codeine is very constipating. His physicians had to periodically re-insert his rectum when it "fell out." He periodically required enemas. Secondly, the combination of oral aspirin, phenacetin, and caffeine at high dosages caused periodic ulceration and bleeding in his stomach. Due to so much blood loss, he even required blood transfusions to raise his hemoglobin to safe levels. The third major problem with his treatment is that excess diazepam (Valium®) is now well known to cause poor balance and frequent falls that may result in a fractured hip. This happened to Hughes and more information about his hip fracture is detailed in the chapter on "Final Years." Dr. Crane initially prescribed diazepam for insomnia and PAT, but it proved to provide some pain relief and control of his OCD and TBI symptoms. HH therefore tried to augment the inadequate pain control provided by codeine compound, so he sometimes took too many diazepam dosages and suffered the complications of oversedation and falls.

Codeine is still used today but only for short-term pain relief. In Hughes' days there was no concept about short or long-acting opioids. Whether an opioid lasts two or six hours depends upon how long it will remain in the blood before the liver deactivates it and the kidneys excrete it. Codeine only lasts about two or three hours. This means that HH had to take a lot of dosages to get 24 hours of pain relief, and this is precisely what he did. His physicians just thought he was abusing codeine by observing his frequent dosing. He was trying to get good pain relief which probably did not occur very often. Nevertheless, he managed somehow to make codeine compound work for 30 years.

Today, HH would be given a longer acting opioid so he would not have to take a pain reliever so frequently. Diazepam (Valium®) has been an enduring drug and is still used for specific purposes such as muscle spasms, tremors, anxiety, and sleep, but usually less than the dosages used by Hughes. As this book is being written a lot of new therapies for IPS are being investigated and implemented. There have been many advances in pain management since the codeine-Valium® days of HH. For example, the first preferred drug for IPS is usually a non-opioid called naltrexone. The first choice of opioid is usually a non-sedating, hard to abuse opioid called buprenorphine. Valium® has been pretty much replaced by a class of drugs which pain-treatment physicians call "neuropathic" as they block painful electric currents in nerves. There are now effective non-opioid pain relievers including ketamine, ketorolac, oxytocin, and cannabinoid products. Other therapies include biochemical surrogates, hormone restoration, and electromagnetic therapies. Persons with the most severe cases of IPS have access to implanted electrical stimulators and opioid administration devices that pump opioids directly into the spinal fluid. Simply put, "we've come a long way" since the days of HH. That said, however, his physicians and aides humanely exploited the best treatments available in the days of HH. They did their best to help Howard live 30 years after he miraculously survived his 1946 airplane crash.

9. Life Extension and Career Change: 1961-1973

""Valium® and a Change of Life"

Heading into the last 15 years of HH's 30-year post-crash survival he suffered from a combination of (1) obsessive-compulsive disorder (OCD), (2) traumatic brain injury (TBI), and (3) intractable pain syndrome (IPS). Partial deafness undoubtedly complicated his overall medical condition. What is critical about understanding the medical saga of HH is that none of his three serious conditions were understood or hardly recognized by the medical profession in 1961. Consequently, the physicians for HH could only provide symptomatic care and curtail complications of his diseases and the medications prescribed to him. For example, they could suppress pain, transfuse blood, and drain pressure sores (decubiti), but they did not fully understand why these medical problems developed. Despite their lack of understanding of HH's basic diseases, they quickly tackled every medical complication and event that occurred. They were extremely frustrated with HH's refusal to obtain medical tests and x-rays, reduce his codeine use, and attempt healing measures such as walking, physical therapy and dental care. Nevertheless, they helped him live 30 years after a near death plane crash which left him seriously injured and in daily pain.

Dr. Norman Crane took over from Dr. Vern Mason the medical care of HH in 1961. More than any other doctor, he cared for HH in his years of deterioration. He had already written prescriptions in the late 1950's for HH as he was the office partner of Dr. Vern Mason who did most of HH's medical care since 1932 and in the first 15 years of HH's post-crash survival. Dr. Mason left the direct care of HH in 1960 when he moved to Miami to supervise the research of the Howard Hughes Medical Institute.

Dr. Crane was officially hired as HH's personal physician on December 1, 1961. His contract specified that he was to give personal attention to HH over his regular medical practice. HH still lived primarily in LA, at the time, and Dr. Crane had his private practice in LA. He continued to be HH's primary doctor after HH moved into the Desert Inn in Las Vegas in 1966 and in other hotels and countries in which HH lived until 1973. At the time he became HH's personal physician in 1961, Dr. Crane testified under oath in the United States versus Thain trial in 1978 that the only drug HH was regularly taking at that time was oral codeine compound (Empirin®). Although Dr. Crane was the primary physician for HH in the 12 years between 1961-1973 he consulted with a few other physicians about specific clinical problems. Dr. Homer Clark, a hematologist and internist, became a second attending physician to HH in 1970. Clark was initially hired primarily to help with transfusing blood for anemia that HH developed due to a bleeding ulcer. Dr. Wilbur Thain took over as primary physician in 1973 after HH had fractured his hip while in a London hotel. Dr. Crane stayed on as one of four attending MD's to HH until Hughes died in 1976. Dr. Crane wrote all HH's medical prescriptions between 1961 and 1973 when Dr. Thain took over prescription writing. Shortly after diazepam (Valium®) came onto the commercial market in 1963, Dr. Crane started HH on it for insomnia and control of PAT.

Interestingly, diazepam (Valium®) appeared to significantly decrease, but not eliminate, his germaphobia and other symptoms of OCD and TBI. He had fewer mental lapses and his thinking improved. These reports are not surprising as the class of drugs called benzodiazepines to which diazepam (Valium®) belongs have been used since about 1964 for a wide variety of mental and physical maladies that affect the CNS.

In 1961 and 1962, Dr. Crane made a medical decision that later confounded all parties, including this author, who attempted to understand why needles were imbedded in HH's arms at his autopsy. These were identified by x-rays which are shown in this book. Dr. Crane taught HH how to inject codeine rather than take it all by mouth. Until then HH had only used oral codeine compound since he left Good Samaritan Hospital in 1946. His oral tablet intake normally varied from 5 to 25 tablets a day and even up to 30 or 40 on days of severe pain flares. Dr. Crane wanted to reduce his oral use of codeine compounds because (1) phenacetin was starting to be recognized as a cause of kidney toxicity (2) aspirin in excessive amounts would cause a peptic ulcer, and (3) caffeine would raise his heart rate and cause PAT with a pulse rate up to 200 beats per minute while the normal rate is about 72 beats per minute. Dr. Crane taught HH how to inject plain codeine phosphate to try to reduce his use of oral codeine compound. Interestingly, HH found that oral codeine compound gave him more "lift" and pain relief than plain injectable codeine. Against medical advice, he would sometimes dissolve codeine compound tablets and inject them. Codeine compound given by injection was fraught with hazards. In those days, injections had to be given with a glass syringe and stainless-steel needle which was not always secure on the syringe and would lodge in tissues. To keep infection down, syringes and needles had to be washed and sterilized. The hygiene of the needles and syringes were left to the aides of HH, so the sterility level of their efforts is uncertain. Some needles HH injected came loose from the syringe and lodged in his arms. Sometimes they would work their way to the surface on their own rather than require surgical incision to remove them. Five needles were left lodged in his arms for an unknown period as evidenced by x-rays taken at autopsy. When observers, such as this author, saw these x-rays, it was assumed that the lodged needles were part of a heinous addiction with illegal opioids since there was no real knowledge of HH's medical condition prior to his autopsy. The decision of Dr. Crane to provide codeine by injection and reduce HH's oral intake of phenacetin and aspirin probably extended HH's life by a few years. This supposition cannot be proved, but the use of injectable codeine likely minimized phenacetin dosage and slowed progression of kidney failure and decreased aspirin use decreased internal bleeding.

Codeine in its various forms and diazepam are the only drugs known to be regularly prescribed by Dr. Crane from 1961 through 1973. Dr. Crane related to me that HH mentally functioned quite well but had slow but definite progressive physical deterioration after 1961. HH managed his own affairs and was always lucid until a few days before his death in 1976. He had strange working habits in that he would work long hours followed by long hours of sleep. He would eat one meal a day which did not necessarily correspond to normal breakfast, lunch, or dinner times. HH did not choose to walk much after 1961 due to pain generated by the painful arthropathies and neuropathies in his hips and legs that were sequelae from his plane crash injuries of 1946. His neck began to be progressively fixated in a leaning forward position. His balance also slowly deteriorated, and he had an unknown number of falls.

In November 1966 HH made some life changing decisions. First, he temporarily moved from LA to Boston where he stayed in the Ritz-Carlton Hotel for about nine days. A rumor was propagated that he was going to Boston to seek help at the Peter Bent Brigham Hospital which was associated with Harvard Medical School. Whether this happened is doubtful. There is no verified report that he went near a doctor in Boston. Even if he had gone to seek medical care, it is doubtful that anyone knew enough in the 1960's about HH's three major disorders that they could provide any better care than what Dr. Crane was doing. There is an undocumented story that he had a Harvard nutritionist design a vitamin and herbal concoction that he could take. When Dr. Thain took over as head physician in 1973, HH was taking a vitamin preparation. He wanted Dr. Thain to explain its benefits. Dr. Thain was not sure what the vitamin preparation was, but thought it was Theragram-M.

HH left Boston after about nine days and traveled by train to Las Vegas. On November 27, 1966 he arrived in Las Vegas and moved into the top floor of the Desert Inn. He had visionary plans to turn the shoddy gambling town into a mecca of recreation. He also saw his Las Vegas as a "center of scientific research and space-age industry, with a new airport, the first in the world designed specifically to accommodate supersonic planes." Indeed, his vision, plus his casino, hotel and land acquisitions in the 1960's certainly laid a foundation for today's Las Vegas.

While living in the top floor of the Desert Inn, HH recruited around-the-clock aides. Although all were male, they functioned as nursing and administrative aides to HH. Some had previous medical experience. They did all his medical needs including food arrangements, bathing, and toiletry. They would assist the doctors when they attended. As HH became less and less agile they would even carry him to a chair, adjust his bed, and facilitate film screening and business communications. By his actions HH clearly intended to live out his life in a hotel setting as he had no immediate family or home residence. Even more critical he became debilitated enough by the mid-1960's that he required the same supportive medical care and services that are found in today's assisted living or nursing home facilities.

HH's decision to move to and re-create Las Vegas is remarkable in that he was quite ill and impaired. He was 61 years old, an age that most persons are choosing a retirement and kick-back lifestyle. Although I have not found any documented statements by HH or his physicians, he must have developed some internal motivation despite his health issues to take on a new career and move his residence. This move and life-change is quite surprising since he was partially deaf, unable to ambulate very well, in constant pain, taking daily opioids, and still fighting imaginary and non-existent germs. He was also impotent and unable to have a marital relationship. It is likely that diazepam (Valium®) helped him stabilize his OCD and TBI symptoms, so he could mentally function well enough to make this significant and positive life change.

During the time of Dr. Crane's care, HH functioned aggressively to expand his businesses and political influence. Much of his activity is legendary and well described in several excellent books. Here is a short list of his business deals to emphasize that he functioned relatively well on his treatment program of codeine and Valium®. He sold RKO Productions which netted $25 million. In 1966 he sold his 6.5 million shares of TWA stock that netted him $546 million. With all the cash he generated on these sales, he was in good financial shape to start his new career in Las Vegas. He purchased many properties in Las Vegas and Nevada including ranch and mining properties and several casinos and hotels including the New Frontier, Sands, Silver Slipper, Castaways, and Harold's Club in Reno He purchased the hotel in which he lived, The Desert Inn. He also purchased Air West Airlines in 1970 which was primarily based in Las Vegas.

On Thanksgiving Eve 1970, HH left Las Vegas, the Desert Inn, and the United States. A long-time friend, Jack Real, flew him to the Bahamas where Howard took up new quarters in the Britannia Beach Hotel. His aides and the support system he developed in Las Vegas, including his physicians, followed him. The usual reason given for his departure from Las Vegas was legal problems with the Federal Internal Revenue Service, civil lawsuits, and federal indictments. Apparently, no new health issue caused him to leave the USA and spend the rest of his life outside the country. HH lived a phantom life after Las Vegas, and he established his own medical abode in whatever swank hotel in which he lived. His doctors brought medical care and medications to him regardless of the hotel or country in which he lived. Other than a few hours plane layover in Miami, HH did not return to the United States until his death in April 1976.

Two major medical events occurred during the care of Dr. Crane. In 1970 HH developed severe anemia and pneumonia. Dr. Crane prescribed effective antibiotics which saved HH. He almost died but was adequately treated by Dr. Crane with the assistance of Dr. Homer Clark who was a hematologist based in Salt Lake City, Utah. Although no laboratory hemoglobin or hematocrit blood levels are known, Dr. Clark flew blood from Salt Lake City to Nassau, Bahamas to transfuse HH. At least one more transfusion was necessary. The cause of the anemia was a bleeding peptic ulcer due to the continuous use of oral codeine which contained aspirin, phenacetin, and caffeine. Both aspirin and phenacetin at high dosages can cause gastric ulcers and bleeding. Clearly, Drs. Crane and Clark saved the life of HH.

The overall health of HH declined between 1960 and 1970, although many of his OCD and TBI symptoms decreased. He was about 15 to 25 years post-crash and his disorders, including deafness, OCD, TBI, and IPS, were taking their toll. At some point in the four years HH lived in Las Vegas between 1966 and 1970 Jean Peters reported that he was not feeling well and that he contemplated returning to LA from Las Vegas for medical treatment. She was not sure exactly what was wrong with him. Mentally, she believed he was all there, despite the fact she believed he was taking too much codeine. She quoted, "I knew he didn't eat correctly. He didn't exercise, and his whole lifestyle had ruined what was once a magnificent physique." In January 1970, the news broke that Jean Peters was leaving HH. Her official public announcement was short and not very explanatory, "This is not a decision made in haste, and is done only with the greatest of regret. Our marriage has endured for thirteen years, which is long by present standards. Any property settlement will be resolved primarily between us." Exactly when Peters last saw HH is unclear. It is known that they had not been living together for an unknown number of years.

Another serious medical incident occurred in 1973 when HH fell and fractured his hip while staying in London. His hip was pinned in a London hospital. Hughes left the hospital within two days after the surgery. He never walked again and was bed-bound until death. Older persons (Hughes was 67) often fall due to drug use with sedatives such as Valium®. Sedating drugs may cause falls because older persons may have loss of balance and weak legs, ankles, or feet. It was after this incident that Bill Gay, Chief of Operations of the Summa Corporation, made Dr. Wilbur Thain the personal physician of HH. He remained head physician between 1973 and the death of HH in 1976. More details on the fall and hip surgery in London the details are found in the chapter "The End Time Years."

Dr. Crane and the other physicians had to care for several complications of his basic diseases and the complications of high dosages of codeine. This included constipation and rectal prolapse. Codeine is notorious for causing severe constipation. His day and night biologic pattern known as circadian rhythm was off. He would often be awake at night and sleep in the daytime. This complication is common with TBI and IPS. Since he could not ambulate well, he spent a lot of time in bed and developed bed sores known as decubiti. Painful urination due to prostatitis was sometimes a problem. A summary of these issues is listed in the accompanying Table.

During the years that Dr. Crane helped care for HH as his primary or attending physician, he kept no records of either medical care, drug prescribing, or administration of drugs. Dr. Crane temporarily stopped giving HH codeine in 1970 because he felt HH had escalated his dose to an unacceptable level. Dr. Crane also believed that he did not need a dose of 15 to 30 grains of codeine a day to control whatever pain he had. The stoppage lasted about four months and then was resumed. It is unknown whether complete stoppage occurred or whether Hughes obtained codeine from other sources. Given the severity of his condition total stoppage was unlikely. Despite a lack of records Dr. Crane provided much needed medical care (see Table). In 1978, Dr. Crane was federally indicted for supplying HH with controlled drugs without proper records that supported a legitimate medical reason for supplying the drugs. He pled "no contest" and, at age 73, he was placed on federal probation. He appeared in the United States versus Thain trial and gave ample reason why HH had serious medical conditions that justified codeine and diazepam (Valium®). Dr. Crane did not enter prison but retired and died in obscurity.

Just why Dr. Crane was replaced by Dr. Thain in 1973 as head physician to HH is not known. One thing is clear. Dr. Norman Crane pulled HH through 12 years of serious medical crises and deterioration. Dr. Crane's indictment unfortunately obscured the fact that he clearly saved HH's life during severe episodes of pneumonia and internal bleeding. He also probably prolonged his life by his decisions to start diazepam (Valium®) and injectable codeine. The change of life that HH made in 1966, at age 61, to essentially start a new career in Las Vegas despite his serious illnesses occurred during Dr. Crane's care. This endeavor must be recognized as an extraordinary deep-seated desire to live and follow a vision. Dr. Crane was a supporter of HH's decision to move to Las Vegas and his approval was probably a boost for Howard because he certainly needed a caring doctor to support his life-changing transition.

MEDICAL ISSUES AND CONDITIONS
OBSERVED BETWEEN 1961 AND 1976

Insomnia
Paroxysmal
Atrial Tachycardia
Deafness
Constipation
Anemia
Peptic Ulcer
Hesitant/Seldom Ambulation
Irregular Dietary Schedule
Bed Sores-Decubiti
Painful Urination (Dysuria)
Rectal Prolapse
Fractured Hip
Fixated Neck
Pain - Multiple Sites
Pneumonia

10. The Activity Logs: Oct. 31, 1971-July 1973

"An Insight to a Hotel Life"

Essentially no standard medical records were ever kept by HH's physicians or were ever released to the public. An unusual set of records, however, were kept which has helped dissect and piece together the medical saga of HH. Between October 31, 1971 and July 1, 1973, the aides of HH kept 244 daily logs of his activities. HH was 66 to 68 years old during this period and he resided in various hotels in multiple countries. The log was typed on legal size paper and simply labeled "log." It is unknown if any other daily logs or records were ever kept by HH's aides. The reason this log was kept is unclear, but they provide a "picture window" into how HH lived and what he did on a day-to-day basis. It supports information provided by his physicians and the findings of his autopsy. Consequently, some pages of the "log" that show specific examples of his activities are published verbatim in the Appendix of this book. The format and style are retained in the samples shown in the Appendix. The log details the specific time of each day that HH engaged in various activities including the following: used toilet, dined, watched films or television, sat in a chair to read, took drugs, transacted business, left the hotel, or was attended by his physicians.

The logs show that HH consumed chicken as his main dietary food. He also ate dessert either alone or with his chicken. Desserts were listed usually as tarts with napoleon cream. On rare occasions he ate beef. He did not eat on a regular schedule but did eat every day. Codeine was not consumed daily, but in exceptionally large doses when it was taken. It was usually consumed as codeine compound. On many days during this period he consumed, in one dose, 10 or 12 codeine which is 600 to

720mg. One notation indicates he consumed 25 codeine (1500mg) in one dose. These doses indicate tremendous tolerance and considerable previous consumption of codeine since single doses of about 800 mg have been fatal in a normal human. His irregular pattern of codeine use is not the usual pattern of opioid addiction which requires daily use. He extensively used diazepam (Valium®), 10mg, and HH's aides referred to them in the log as BB's "Blue Bombers" since they are a blue tablet. HH would often consume four or five (40-50 mg) at a time, usually to sleep. Some days he consumed as many as nine tablets (90mg) of Valium® which indicates considerable tolerance to this drug and long-term previous consumption. The log indicates that HH's aides and doctors did several personal care duties. They changed bandages on his bed sores and picked him up from at least two falls including one when he fell off the toilet. They occasionally trimmed his hair, beard, and nails but there is no mention of tooth brushing or cleaning. Beginning on June 14, 1972 there are notations that Hughes required the "Big E" which was an enema.

The log indicates that HH could mentally function well at least intermittently during this period. HH transacted some business, including stock sales, leases, and tax decisions. He met with President Somoza of Nicaragua on March 13, 1972. On at least one occasion he left his hotel to fly a plane. He frequently read newspapers. The log also recounts the famous telephone interview on January 7, 1972, regarding the fraudulent Clifford Irving biography. He made several trips and stayed in numerous locations, including Managua, Vancouver, and London, England.

During the 20 months this log was kept, it shows that he "screened" 530 different movies. Some were repeatedly watched. The most watched was "Jungle," 16 times, and "Shanghai Express," 14 times. There are notes in the log to send the films "back" with or without his approval. For example, he did not like "Ghost Train," but really liked "Bedford Incident." Of interest is that there was a torture scene about ½ way through the "Ipcress File" that he did not want to see. He had his aides stop the film before this scene appeared. It is unclear from the log as to whether his almost daily screening of films was purely for his entertainment or whether his "approval" had some business or potential business ramification since the word "screen" is used rather than just "watch" or "view."

The log was abruptly discontinued when he fell and fractured his hip in London on July 1, 1973. It is clear in the log that HH had good control of his mental faculties and seemed in firm control of all his various activities during this time-period, 1971 to 1973. The kind of medical care he received appeared typical of what a 66 to 68-year-old person would receive in a nursing home or assisted living facility.

Above all, the logs show that he received reasonably good custodial and nursing care with diet, medication, sanitation, and assistance with ambulation since he could not walk well due to his injuries and progressive neurological impairments. Perhaps a description could have been purposely left off the log, but there is no mention of episodes of psychosis or germ avoidance. It was clear that his OCD was still with him, however, because he repeatedly watched some films a considerable number of times. It also appears that his medications, codeine, and diazepam (Valium®), were helping him as there is no mention of memory loss, hiding from staff, performing a spectacle such as repetitive note writing, or making a paranoid claim about persons or events. These were all done when he was younger when he had no benefit of medications.

11. The Aviator's Last Flights: May 12, 1973

""An End of Life Wish is Accomplished"

As sick as he was during the last years of his life, HH had a dream to fly one more time before he died. In his last few years of life, he had a close friend and confidant, Jack Real, who was an expert pilot and helped HH with various needs. He arranged for the first of his last flights in London on May 12, 1973. Real arranged for HH to "test fly" a brand-new Hawker-Siddeley 748, a hefty, twin-engine turboprop. Tony Blackman, the chief test pilot for Hawker-Siddeley, agreed to serve as copilot for obvious reasons. HH had not flown a plane for over 25 years and was on an opioid for his painful condition. Also, his legs did not flex very well.

On the morning of May 12, 1973 HH joyously made his way into the lobby of the London Inn dressed in new clothes clutching his new lucky fedora. No wonder. He had miraculously survived four plane crashes wearing his famous fedora. He did not appear drugged but was totally lucid, talkative, and appeared to be a professional flyer. From a medical perspective an unusual event occurred. After he entered the cockpit of the aircraft, he shed his light blue shirt, unzipped, and took off his slacks and dropped his drawstring shorts. Naked and smiling he wore his fedora, eased into the pilot's seat, fired up the engines and taxied down the runway. He not only flew flawlessly on this trip he did three more flights between May and July 1973. One of them was across the English Channel to Ostend, Belgium.

The sight of removal of his trousers and underwear must have been a bizarre experience for his copilot and even Jack Real. Little did they know that HH's IPS condition can make it impossible to tolerate the pain brought on by mere underwear and regular clothes. There is no record of HH discussing this unusual and rare pain sensitivity to anyone other than his physicians. This is not uncommon in persons who develop IPS to have severe allodynia (skin sensitivity). Few persons will discuss it out of embarrassment or fear of being labeled psychotic. The fact that he could still pilot an airplane at age 68 with his horrific medical conditions is a tribute to the medical and custodial care that he received in his chosen, reclusive lifestyle in luxury hotels.

12. The End-Time Years: 1973-1976

"Doctors Prolong His Life"

In early 1972 Frank William Gay (Bill), the Chief Executive of the Hughes Nevada Empire asked Wilbur Thain, MD if he would be available to see HH for "some medical problems." At the time Dr. Thain had a private, active family practice in Logan, Utah. Interestingly, Bill Gay was a brother-in-law to Dr. Thain having married his sister.

In 1972, the attending physicians for HH were Drs. Norman Crane and Homer Clark. It is uncertain why Bill Gay wanted Dr. Thain to see HH, but at age 67 he was having multiple health issues and was in the late stages of his life. In August of 1972, Bill Gay asked Dr. Thain to spend two weeks in Vancouver, British Columbia with HH. Thain was booked with his own practice, but he went to Vancouver for five days and never saw HH. When Dr. Thain landed, Dr. Clark was leaving Vancouver. On his way to the airport, he informed Dr. Thain about two recurrent health issues that would require immediate attention when they occurred: (1) paroxysmal atrial tachycardia (PAT) and rectal prolapse. Thain made a second short trip to Vancouver in September 1972 but again did not see HH.

After his second trip to Vancouver, which Bill Gay arranged in December 1972, a regular eight-week rotation was devised for the three physicians who would attend HH: Dr. Crane, Dr. Clark, and Dr. Thain. The initial rotation was two weeks each for Dr. Thain and Dr. Clark and four weeks for Dr. Crane.

The first time that Dr. Thain saw HH was in May 1973 while HH was staying in London. At the time Dr. Crane briefed Dr. Thain on his major concerns regarding the health of HH: (1) anemia with possible carcinoma of stomach, (2) multiple pain complaints, (3) poor eating habits, (4) constipation, and (5) dental hygiene with refusal to see a dentist or brush his teeth. Dr. Crane also informed Dr. Thain that they had on hand physical examination equipment including a stethoscope and blood pressure cuff. There was a centrifuge, dipsticks, and microscope to do urinalyses as well as an electrocardiogram. Dr. Crane informed Dr. Thain that frequent urinalysis had all been normal. Interestingly, the first face-to-face visit between Dr. Thain and HH was to discuss the multiple vitamin/mineral preparation that HH was taking. Dr. Thain later related in his trial that the preparation was probably "Theragram-M." HH reviewed every mineral and vitamin and wanted to know, in detail, why he needed them and what they would do for him. Dr. Thain reported that HH was very lucid and communicative. HH also remembered that Dr. Thain had worked for the Hughes Company as an administrative aide between 1948 and 1952 before Dr. Thain went to medical school.

In the May 1973 meeting Dr. Thain described HH as alert, facultative, and thin weighing about 130 pounds. His hair had grown to shoulder length and he had grown a beard whereas in 1948-52 Dr. Thain recalled he only had worn a mustache. Dr. Thain did notice a lump of fibrous scar tissue on the top of his head, but he did not discuss it with Howard.

The next visit to HH was August 10, 1973 where HH was staying at the Inn-on-the-Park Hotel in London. When Dr. Thain arrived, he was informed by aides that HH had fallen in the bathroom on August 9. HH was put back in bed, and Dr. Clark did not believe there was any significant damage due to the fall. Dr. Thain examined HH and found that he was in bed with his knee bent and hip rotated to the outside. Dr. Thain believed he had a fractured hip, so he contacted a British doctor, Arthur Levin. After hearing that Dr. Thain believed HH had a fractured hip, Dr. Levin arranged for an x-ray unit to be brought to the hotel room of HH. An x-ray did show a fracture of the hip. There was no displacement of the hip which made surgery less problematic. Dr. Thain and a British radiologist, Dr. Young, informed HH that he would have to go into a hospital to have his hip pinned by a competent orthopedic surgeon. HH tried to resist but finally agreed to the surgery in a hospital.

On August 10, 1973, HH was admitted to the London Hospital under an assumed name. At that time British hospitals often used assumed names for famous people. In the hospital Dr. Thain was able to perform a physical exam on HH while he was under pentothal anesthetic just before the surgery. His blood pressure was 124 over 72. Respirations were 20 per minute. His heart, lungs, abdomen, and prostate were normal. He had some hemorrhoids. Peripheral pulses in his legs and neck were normal.

Interestingly, HH informed Dr. Thain just before surgery that he was taking 25 to 40 grains of codeine a day. HH was worried that his codeine use might interfere or be toxic with the surgical anesthetic. The surgery itself took about 70 minutes and was expertly done by Sir Walter Robinson, a noted British orthopedist. The day after surgery HH returned to his hotel. On the next day he was recovering well with a slight temperature. HH was given antibiotics and pain from the hip resolved.

Dr. Thain left for the States on August 18, 1973 as he was relieved by Dr. Lawrence Chaffin who was summoned to help with surgical matters including HH's post-operative care and bed sores (decubiti). Other than a one to two-day short trip to London, in November 1973, Dr. Thain did not see HH for the next year until August of 1974.

In December 1973, HH moved from London to the Xanadu Hotel in Freeport, Bahamas. Dr. Thain traveled to Freeport in April 1974 for his regular rotation but apparently did not personally see HH until August of 1974. On April 26, 1974, Dr. Crane informed Dr. Thain that he was going to stop writing all prescriptions of codeine and Valium® for Mr. Hughes. Dr. Thain was, therefore, appointed head physician by Bill Gay. HH's medication dosages at that time were about 25 to 40 grains a day of codeine and 7 to 15, 10 milligram Valium® a day. Given Dr. Crane's desire to cease prescribing and what both doctors believed to be excessive daily dosages of codeine and diazepam, they had a seven-hour meeting with HH on August 3, 1974. HH was 68 years old. In the meeting HH was quite talkative, alert, and told many stories about his childhood and love for Jean Peters. The purpose of the meeting was to put HH on a withdrawal program that would have him off all drugs by December 24, 1974 which was his birthday. Howard, in the meeting, told the physicians that he could get by on 10 to 12 grains of codeine a day. Dr. Crane and Dr. Thain agreed to give HH six, 10 mg Valium® a week principally for sleep. Dr. Thain worked out a straight-line withdrawal schedule for codeine and put the amounts in envelopes to be given to HH each week and in a manner that would ensure that he was totally off codeine in the week before December 24, 1974. The doctor on duty would give HH his weekly allotment. Besides reducing the amount of codeine each week, Dr. Thain tried to substitute codeine with Tylenol®, placebos, and plain codeine to reduce the amount of phenacetin that HH had been taking. Unfortunately, codeine with Tylenol® was not highly effective and HH complained bitterly about the re-emergence of severe pain in his neck, back, and hips. By December 1974 it became obvious that HH could not totally stop codeine. Consequently, Dr. Thain drastically reduced, but continued giving HH codeine and Valium® until his death in April 1976. In the 18 months between November 1974 and his death in early April 1976, Dr. Thain gave HH 48 codeine tablets and six Valium® tablets per week. This was a codeine dose of about 6.8 grains per day and represented a major, approximately 50% codeine reduction in daily dosage and an 80-90% reduction in daily dosage of Valium®, since Hughes was previously taking 40 to 50 Valium® a week. Unfortunately, the great reduction of codeine and Valium® in the 18 months before HH died had a real downside. Unknown to his doctors HH started a major usage of Excedrin®. This non-prescription drug which HH acquired through unknown sources contained a combination of aspirin, acetaminophen, salicylamide, and caffeine. Dr. Thain informed HH that he should limit his daily intake of Excedrin® to 12 a day. As with all intractable pain patients who cannot obtain their preferred and effective pain reliever, however, HH resorted to the only drug he could obtain while bed-bound and in a hotel - Excedrin®. Unfortunately, he did not limit his intake to 12 a day. HH took up to 20 tablets a day. Aspirin and its related compound, salicylamide, at this dosage is simply too much for human tissues to tolerate. The autopsy of HH showed he had an on-going peptic ulcer in the stomach and two forms of renal disease: interstitial fibrosis due to phenacetin and papillary necrosis or disintegration (tips of kidney tubule) from excess aspirin and salicylates. There was a major unintended consequence of the physician's desire to lower HH's daily codeine and Valium® dosages. HH began to substitute Excedrin® in such excess amounts that it likely hastened his death by some unknown period of time.

13. Final Four Days: April 3-7, 1976

"Kidneys Fail Due to Phenacetin"

In the 18 months between November 1974 and April 1976, HH's physicians felt they had achieved a milestone in limiting his codeine and Valium®. Little did they know of HH's excessive Excedrin® use and that high dose Excedrin® was causing a little more kidney tissue to dissolve each day. On Saturday, April 3, 1976, HH was living in the penthouse suite, 20th floor of the Acapulco, Mexico, Princess Hotel. He suddenly, without much warning slipped into a "trance-like state."

HH's aide on duty on this day, George Francom, recognized that HH was not verbally responding and appeared to have deteriorated. HH also did not have a reaction when Francom waved a hand in front of his face. Francom summoned Dr. Lawrence Chaffin who was the physician on duty. Dr. Chaffin quickly recognized impending coma and contacted the hotel's local doctor, Victor Manuel Montemayor, to assist in obtaining a blood test to determine the cause. Diabetes was suspected but the glucose blood level was reportedly 122 (normal is about 80 to 120) which ruled out diabetic coma. Unexpectedly the blood urea nitrogen usually called BUN was 104.5mg (normal is about 20-40mg). This was unexpected by Dr. Chaffin because HH never allowed any blood tests to tip off his physicians that his kidneys were failing. The last and apparently the only blood tests HH had in the last 30 years of his life were done in a London Hospital in 1973 when he fractured his hip which required pinning. At this time, his BUN was normal.

After learning about what appeared to be kidney failure and what is known as "uremic poisoning," Dr. Chaffin contacted HH's other two physicians, Drs. Norman Crane, and Wilbur Thain. A collective decision was made to try and get HH to the nearest hospital that would have emergency kidney dialysis and other high-tech capability. The hotel doctor, Victor Manuel Montemayor, informed Hughes' doctors that the type of upscale medical treatment to save Hughes was not available in Mexico. A plane was enlisted and a flight to Houston to secure help at its famous Methodist Hospital was arranged. On April 5, 1976, at 11:00 AM, HH along with Drs. Thain and Chaffin and aide John Holmes boarded the plane for the flight from Acapulco to Houston.

The doctors fully realized that HH was near death and did everything that doctors normally do to possibly save a life that is close to terminus. An intravenous drip was started to boost hydration and HH was put in a closed oxygen tent. He had some seizures and was given intravenous corticosteroids to possibly prevent cerebral edema. Despite these efforts HH died on the plane at 1:27 PM.

The aircraft carrying HH, and his physicians touched down about 2:00 PM approximately 30 minutes after Dr. Thain had pronounced him dead. Methodist Hospital was well prepared to provide emergency care had HH still been alive. They had received a call earlier that morning from the Miami-based Hughes Medical Institute asking that the hospital be prepared to provide emergency care for HH. Methodist was one of 12 US institutions that were receiving financial support from the Institute. Apparently, the hospital had the initial belief that HH was in diabetic coma, as diabetic and uremic coma appear clinically quite similar and are sometimes only distinguished by blood tests. It is unknown exactly who asked the Institute to call Methodist Hospital or precisely what medical information was transmitted.

Henry D. McIntosh M.D. was chief of the medical service at Methodist and Jack L Titus M.D., PhD, was head of pathology. Methodist Hospital was affiliated with the Baylor College of Medicine. These gentlemen decided that they would not alter the confidentiality or ethics normally applied to a normal, non-famous person. Consequently, extraordinarily little information was provided about HH's death or autopsy findings by Methodist Hospital. Naturally, media was disappointed, because they felt the public had a right to know about America's richest and most mysterious man.

On April 5 after HH had arrived at Methodist Hospital, the hospital issued only these brief news releases.

1. *"Today at 1:27 PM in route from Acapulco to Houston by air, Mr. Howard R. Hughes expired. Mr. Hughes was en route to the Methodist Hospital for medical treatment."*
2. *"Officials of the Methodist Hospital have consulted with Dr. Joseph Jachimczyk, chief medical examiner, and Dr. Ethel Erickson, deputy medical examiner. Additional information will not be available until consultations with attending physicians are completed sometime tomorrow."*

There was a question as to whether the body was HH, so fingerprints were obtained before starting the autopsy. Security had to be instituted because hospital personnel were clandestinely offered as much as $500,000 to provide a photograph of HH. A technical snag was encountered because the two physicians that accompanied HH, Dr. Thain and Dr. Chaffin, were not licensed in

Texas. Consequently, Texas state law required that the death be reported through the office of the Harris County Medical Examiner, Joseph A. Jachimczyk M.D. Furthermore, an autopsy could not be performed without the permission of next of kin. The next of kin was Mrs. F.R. Lummis Sr., Hughes aunt. She was not immediately available, so the next morning on April 6, 1976, William R. Lummis, on behalf of his mother, Mrs. Lummis gave permission to perform the autopsy.

The autopsy was done the afternoon of April 6, 1976 between 1:30 and 3:10 PM. Dr. Titus was the lead physician in charge. Dr. Titus was assisted by two of Methodist Hospital's senior pathologists. Also attending were Drs. McIntosh, Jachimczyk, Erickson, Thain, and Chaffin. In all, eight physicians attended the autopsy, and all agreed on the findings, a fact disregarded by numerous news articles that followed the final four days. The last official press conference given by Methodist Hospital was at 4:00 PM on April 6 about 30 minutes after the autopsy was finished. The press conference was short, only about 25 minutes in length. The hospital emphasized that they had taken extra efforts to identify HH by fingerprints and dental chart. The autopsy was performed like the 400 to 500 done at the hospital each year. The cause of death was chronic renal disease. The official cause of death was "chronic interstitial nephritis with papillary necrosis."

In a separate statement from the hospital report, Dr. Jachimczyk, the Harris County Medical Examiner, said there was no evidence of foul play. Dr. Jachimczyk stated for the public that HH's preliminary toxicology tests were negative except for the presence of codeine which undoubtedly was used as a therapeutic measure. "There's no question the man was in pain." Dr. Jachimczyk also reported that HH was emaciated and shrunken, the body weighing 90 pounds and looking much like a terminal cancer patient, but that he had no major anatomical abnormalities other than the ravages of chronic renal failure. HH had a moustache, goatee, and long hair. He also said his appearance was not grotesque.

Since no pictures were taken of HH at autopsy, his appearance became a source of great imagination as many drawings were made of HH based mainly on reports of his aides. Many of the drawings are grotesque. There are even reports that one aide cut his toenails and hair before he boarded the plane in route to Houston so he would not look grotesque. These various claims, however, do not have enough credibility to be accepted as fact. As soon as his autopsy was completed on April 6, 1976, he was rushed in a hearse to the George H. Lewis & Sons Funeral Home. He was quickly embalmed. A casket was chosen by his cousin William Rice Lummis who had only met HH when he was a boy. Another Lummis family member bought a blue suit for Howard to wear. While at the funeral home, which was less than 24 hours after the autopsy the home was deluged with calls. Jean Peters was one of the few people who knew HH had died, and she called about services. On April 7, 1976, he was buried in an unmarked grave beside his mother at the historic Houston cemetery, Glenwood. The service was attended by about 20 people including eight surviving cousins and their immediate families. HH had not spoken to most of these people since 1938 at the latest. There were no vestiges of HH's Hollywood life such as the attendance of an actress. There was a 10-minute Episcopal memorial led by Reverend Robert T. Gibson, Dean of Christ Church Cathedral of Houston. He read from Chapter 14 of the Book of John, "We brought nothing into this world, and it is certain we can carry nothing out." These words, unfortunately, did not convey the many contributions that HH left us during his 70 years despite his severe handicaps. Funeral services always recognize the positive benefits that someone gives society during their life. HH's funeral services did not give him a single word of credit for anything.

Press was everywhere at the burial site so the world would know the end had come for a famous man. After the casket was lowered and covered, the flowers came. A striking five-foot high airplane-shaped arrangement of pompoms came from an anonymous

Southern California Fitness Club. It was adorned with a red, white, and blue ribbon that read: “He came, he saw, he conquered.”

There was also a bouquet of red roses sent by an anonymous sender suspected to be Jean Peters. What’s not secret is that Jean Peters continued to decorate his grave for several weeks afterward. At the end of his final four days little was known about his medical saga. Methodist Hospital maintained HH’s confidentiality. The billionaire was truly dead and died of kidney failure. He had been in pain and therapeutically used codeine. Numerous lawsuits and legal challenges, however, after his final four days required release of his autopsy report including toxicologic analysis and x-rays that were given to select parties including this author. An analysis of his autopsy is given here as it confirms and reveals much of HH’s medical saga. For example, after the final four days there was no initial concept that HH’s kidney failure started with a plane crash which occurred 30 years prior.

14. The Autopsy and Toxicology Findings

"Renal Failure and a Codeine Mystery"

Autopsies are done either to confirm an illness that was present during life and/or explain why a death has occurred. The autopsy of HH did both. In HH's case that autopsy confirmed and pinpointed a specific cause of death, and corroborated the clinical care rendered to him. The autopsy and toxicology analysis were performed with the best technology available in April 1976 and was performed by an expert group of pathologists and toxicologists. Eight physicians observed the autopsy. Jack L. Titus, MD, PhD, was the Chief of Pathology Service at Methodist Hospital in Houston and oversaw the autopsy and toxicology process. It is to the great credit of Dr. Jack Titus and Methodist Hospital that they "played it straight" and "by the book." Later the autopsy and toxicology reports generated by Dr. Titus and Methodist Hospital were given to me to help prepare a report for the Federal Government and use it as evidence in the trial to prosecute Dr. Thain. At the time the autopsy and toxicology analysis were done between April 5 and 7, 1976, essentially no information about the health and medical care of HH had been known to the public for almost 30 years. Needless to say, an emaciated, dehydrated elderly man of about 90 pounds with imbedded needles in his arms, codeine in his blood, and death occurring on a plane over the Gulf of Mexico was strange, shocking, and ample to believe that foul play, illegal activity, and opioid addiction were part of the story. Only after extensive medical investigation, the trial of Dr. Thain, and a later understanding of OCD, TBI, and IPS did the autopsy and toxicology analysis make real sense.

Various theories about HH and his life immediately emanated from his autopsy and toxicology analysis. Many news pieces and books reported theories including murder by codeine injection, forcible addiction to manipulate financial decisions, and deprivation of medical care to hasten death. Other reports said HH really did not have pain or a medical disorder. I have read quotes supposedly said by Dr. Titus that are simply contradictory to what was found at autopsy and which he recorded in writing.

To ensure that the facts and history about HH are preserved, I have placed in the appendix, without change or editing, the autopsy protocol, findings, and toxicology report. Also included are Dr. Titus' report to Henry D. McIntosh MD, Chief of Medical Services of Methodist Hospital, and a description of procedures used to legally identify HH and perform his autopsy. Dr. McIntosh summed up the attitude of the medical team and Methodist Hospital regarding HH, *"Howard Hughes had sought privacy and a lifestyle of secrecy while living, in death, he deserves no less."*

Dr. Titus summarized the autopsy and toxicology analysis, *"The anatomic findings combined with the history of prolonged use of phenacetin containing analgesics establish the renal lesion as analgesic nephropathy (see BURR, AF, Nephron 5:185-201, 1967). The recent, two-day premortem and postmortem chemical analysis document impaired renal function. The toxicologic studies show only minimal amounts of codeine and salicylate."*

In Dr. Titus' letter to Dr. McIntosh on April 7, 1976, he listed the cause of death and major diagnoses. Dr. Titus signed the "Certificate of Death" for HH on April 7, 1976. The immediate cause was "chronic renal failure" and due to "chronic interstitial nephritis with papillary necrosis."

There were other findings listed in his letter and the following were added at the end of the physical and microscopic components of the autopsy: scoliosis of the dorsal spine, diverticulosis of the colon, and lipoma of the left upper arm.

The toxicology report showed codeine in body fluids but no phenacetin or acetylsalicylic acid (aspirin). Benzodiazepines were apparently not assayed.

A dental examination was performed by Oscar Maldonado DDS on April 6, 1976 and his report contained this statement: *"Mr. Hughes teeth were in a poor condition of neglect. He had a generalized condition of chronic periodontal disease with inflammation and hypertrophy of his gum tissue. He also had large areas of tartar deposits around his lower anterior teeth. Most of his upper and lower anterior teeth were loose due to the periodontal disease with bone resorption."*

Roentgenograms or x-rays taken during the autopsy proceedings show five needles imbedded in his arms, osteoporosis, collapsed cervical (neck) vertebrae, and scoliosis of the spine.

The toxicology report shows that there was 0.196mg % (milligram) codeine in the blood. This figure became a matter of controversy because Dr. Titus put in writing that this amount was a "minimal" amount. Later, Dr. Titus claimed he misread the report thinking that the 0.196mg % was micrograms rather than milligrams. This was a big difference in that a microgram is 1/1000 of a milligram. Even though Dr. Titus misread or miscalculated the codeine level in his blood, his mistake had no relevance. I calculated that HH had received small or modest amounts of codeine within hours of his death. Given his renal failure, and tolerance to codeine after 30 years of use, it is not possible to know the precise time that codeine was last taken before death or his last dosage of codeine. Dr. Norman Crane gave him an injection of codeine three days before his death. It is unknown how much codeine was given to HH or whether he received additional codeine just prior to death. Regardless, the toxicology analysis determined that the post-mortem codeine levels in his body fluids were not high enough to make any claims of intentional or accidental overdose considering his renal failure and long-term tolerance to codeine.

In summary, HH's autopsy and toxicologic analysis were extensive and the results were recorded in a most straightforward and professional manner. The pathologists and toxicologists had no prior knowledge of his complex medical history, his rare medical disorders, or his clinical care. They did their job extremely well and in such a manner that the findings all make sense now that we understand the three major medical disorders that afflicted HH and the lifestyle he chose and the treatment he received.

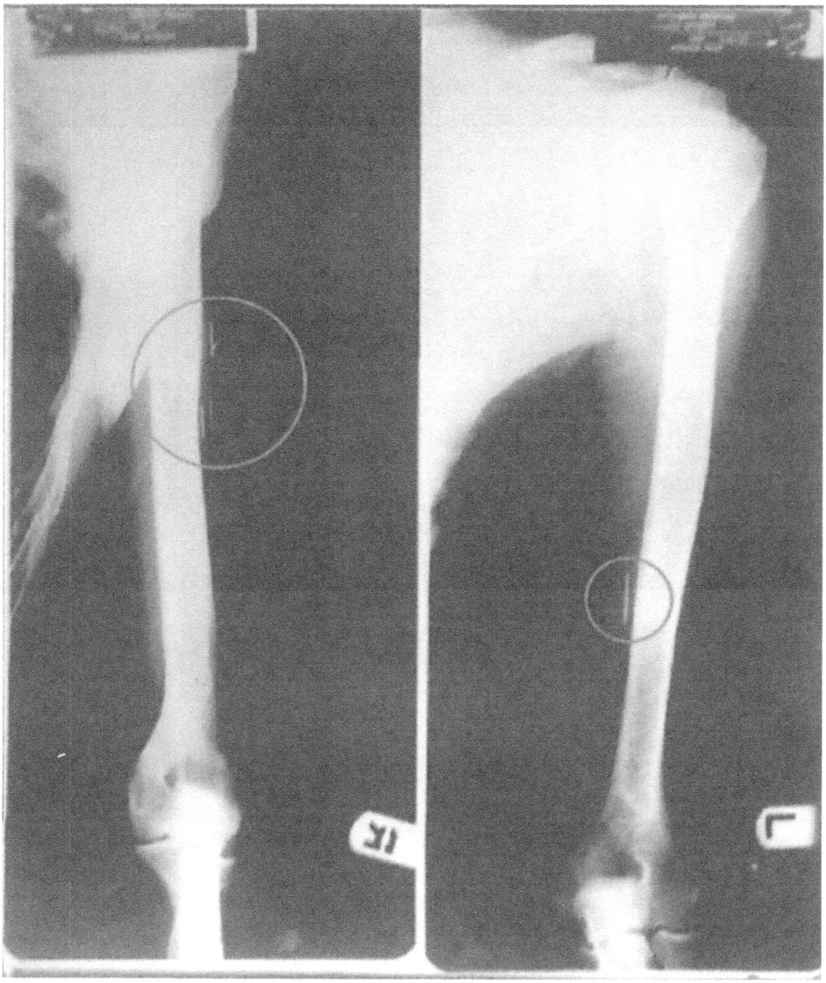

These x-rays taken at autopsy show five needles imbedded in Hughes arms. Hughes had self-injected codeine intramuscularly with outmoded glass syringes that had detachable needles which frequently came loose under the skin.

When these x-rays were first observed, an erroneous conclusion was made that they indicated addiction and abuse rather than a legitimate effort to suppress intractable pain.

15. The Medical Dots All Connect

"History, Medical Cure, and Autopsy all Match Up"

Until recent times the medical history of HH did not make a lot of sense. There were too many holes. His behaviors, autopsy, and medical care seemed disconnected. After all, germaphobia, kidney failure, plane crashes, secretive hideaways, and codeine do not seem to have a connection at first glance. Now that we understand his three major medical conditions – OCD, TBI, and IPS – the dots all connect. His medical saga makes logical sense, and all his bizarre behaviors and symptoms have a reasonable explanation and connection.

His germaphobia, bizarre behaviors, and social isolation were initiated by his two inherited conditions, OCD, and deafness. These disorders were compounded by a rather incredible string of TBI's including at least five that caused unconsciousness. Unfortunately, there was essentially no recognition that OCD and TBI during the lifetime of HH were serious disorders of the CNS that required medical treatment. Even more important is that the combination of both made each more symptomatic. Had there been recognition and treatment of these two conditions as there is today, the medical saga of HH would undoubtedly be quite different. These two disorders caused HH to make some illogical and even dangerous decisions. The most deleterious was his deliberate failure at age 41 to follow the safety protocol for the experimental military reconnaissance plane, the XF-11, in 1946. The crash did not have to occur. The crash of the XF-11 eventually gave him IPS on top of his OCD and TBI. In the relatively rare instance of IPS, severe constant pain produces biochemical changes in the brain that cause endocrine and cardiac dysfunction. He had recurrent episodes of heart racing known as paroxysmal atrial tachycardia (PAT). His autopsy showed enough arteriosclerosis that this condition undoubtedly would have taken his life within a few years if renal failure had not done so. In IPS cortisol is continually raised which causes loss of calcium in bone and teeth. His dental decay, osteoporosis, vertebral collapse, shrunken height, scoliosis, and hip fracture were all undoubtedly related to his IPS and to hormonal abnormalities. Insulin also raises in IPS and accelerates any cholesterol or diabetic tendencies that one may have to form arteriosclerosis. Also, he clearly had testosterone deficiency due to his pain and opioid intake as there are no indications he womanized after about the mid-1950's. Testosterone is necessary in both men and women to build and heal bone, teeth, and other tissues. HH also was averse to any kind of exercise or regular diet. Most physicians, including those of HH, were extremely disappointed in HH's refusal to participate in physical therapy and dental care.

The severe injuries sustained in the 1946 airplane crash required codeine and later diazepam (Valium®) to help control his pain and insomnia. While these two medications helped him make it to age 70, they did not totally control his pain and insomnia. His secretive and reclusive life beginning in the early 1950's at about age 46 appeared to be a combined result of OCD, TBI, and IPS. Reclusiveness probably caused some stress reduction and avoidance, but his three major disorders were progressive, deteriorating conditions that had no known medical treatments at that time in history.

Diazepam (Valium®) came onto the commercial market in 1963 to principally be prescribed for anxiety and stressful situations. It appeared to help control HH's symptoms of OCD and TBI as well as pain. In fact, it may have been enough medical assistance to allow him the mental stability and motivation to make his move to Las Vegas. Much has been written about the appearance of HH during his reclusive, secretive years that he lived in some of the world's luxury hotels. Pictures have been drawn showing him to be a grotesque figure with long hair and fingernails. It is now clearly known that persons with IPS may develop an extreme, painful sensitivity to even light touch. This condition is known as allodynia. Persons with IPS hypersensitivity may experience pain with toothbrushing, hair combing, or nail cutting. Even the touch of clothes may hurt. Both TBI and IPS may cause hypersensitivity to light, some odors, and noise. In summary, all three of his major medical disorders contributed to his reclusiveness and social isolation.

A note is made here of his footwear. He normally had a pair of old soft house shoes or he went barefoot. The pictures and reports of his wearing tissue boxes for shoes is misconstrued. He did wear them one time when his hotel room flooded due to some broken plumbing, but routine use of tissue boxes did not happen. To understand what HH looked like, one should visit a nursing home and look at persons there who have chronic illness and are in their late 60's. No one there will have their previous "Hollywood good looks."

His death in 1976 was not only a shock to the public, but few medical persons at the time were even aware that long-term phenacetin use could cause renal failure. Hughes death made the toxicity of phenacetin a well-known complication, and it was taken off the commercial market a short time after HH's death.

16. Medical Facts Erase Some Myths

"Hughes was Brilliant and Eccentric, and Terribly Ill"

On the day that HH died, myths and theories blossomed like crabgrass and dandelions in Spring. Just like these unwanted visitors, they have been hard to eliminate. The most serious theories suggested heinous and criminal behaviors on the part of HH's company executives, physicians, and close aides. Many parties believed that HH had been a victim of (1) medical neglect, (2) blackmailed by withholding codeine, or (3) murdered with intentional codeine administration.

Medical neglect was theorized to exist because this supposedly would weaken him so he would not make good business decisions or be aware of misuse of company money. Also, neglect might hasten his death. Blackmail by withholding narcotics to an addict is an age-old malignant manipulation to force someone to do something they would not ordinarily do such as steal, have sexual relations, join a gang, or pay money. The high level of codeine in HH's blood at autopsy was believed by some parties to have been put there to murder him and take control of his empire. The physicians most theorized to have been part of the three serious offenses listed above were Drs. Norman Crane and Wilbur Thain. To enhance the theories Dr. Crane pleaded "no contest" in 1978 to charges in a federal indictment that claimed he prescribed controlled drugs to HH without a legitimate medical purpose.

Wilbur Thain, MD was also indicted and charged with prescribing and administering controlled drugs to HH without a legitimate medical purpose, but he highly objected to this charge and decided to challenge the government in court. The trial to prosecute Thain (United States of America versus Wilbur Sutton Thain) was held in the US District Court for the Northern Division of Utah in Ogden, Utah during the week of September 21, 1978. Prior to the trial the US Government and its experts, including this author, clearly believed that Dr. Thain had supplied the controlled drugs codeine and diazepam (Valium®) to a person who was simply an addict with no legitimate medical condition. The reasons for this belief were: (1) autopsy x-rays that showed broken off needles in HH's arms, (2) codeine in his body fluids at the time of death, and (3) an absence of any medical records. The only records available were order blanks for purchase and shipping of drugs. To the great credit of Dr. Thain, he had kept to the surprise of all, detailed records of his care and administration of drugs to HH. Above all he was able to verify that HH had severe arthritis and neuropathic pain in his neck, shoulder, arms, and chest. Autopsy findings supported Dr. Thain's testimony. Other causes of pain were a chronic peptic ulcer, dental decay, and a healed hip fracture. He explained the physician rotation that attended HH even though he was in a foreign country and lived in a luxury hotel. Dr. Chaffin testified to HH's serious injuries and the need for his surgical expertise to treat his bed sores (decubiti), rectal prolapse, and imbedded needles. Even Dr. Crane's testimony acknowledged that HH had serious medical issues despite his "no contest" plea to prescribing codeine and diazepam (Valium®) without a legitimate medical reason. The essence of my medical analysis and report was a theme throughout the trial. Dr. Jack Titus, who performed the autopsy on HH, also testified. He clarified his interpretation of

HH's codeine found in his blood at autopsy as he initially misread the level. Even this clarification did not bring about any new medical interpretation or conclusion, because HH's blood level was compatible with a long-standing codeine tolerance in a person who had renal failure. The jury, after receiving and hearing testimony, acquitted Dr. Thain. Those of us who testified against Dr. Thain and previously believed that some crimes had been committed were somewhat embarrassed, but prior to this trial HH's secretive, out-of-the-country existence and total lack of medical records did not provide us with much information.

Interestingly, about two years after his trial, I was able to personally meet with Dr. Thain at a family practice, post-graduate course in which I was an instructor. We discussed the case of HH, and I congratulated him on his testimony in his trial as well as the care he rendered and the records he kept. Also, I encouraged him to tell his story to Dennis Breo, the expert writer for the American Medical Association. His rendition of his medical care of HH is recorded in a little known but brilliant book entitled "Extra Care." This book has a chapter solely dedicated to the care of HH, and I have literally extracted from it, because it covers the Methodist Hospital autopsy proceedings and Dr. Thain's end-of-life care. Dr. Thain's trial essentially negated any theories of neglected care, blackmail by withholding codeine, and murder by codeine administration.

HH began regular codeine administration in 1946 immediately after he left the hospital for his lifesaving treatment due to his air crash injuries. About one week just prior to his death, he became solemn and unresponsive to verbal inquiry. This is typical of kidney failure. When kidneys start to fail a toxic biochemical called urea-nitrogen begins to back up in the blood and cloud the brain. The kidneys are comprised of filters called glomeruli. They can function and filter out urea-nitrogen even if 80 to 90% of the filters are diseased and eroded. When only a few filters are left intact, however, urea nitrogen is not eliminated. Death comes when the last filters cease to function. HH was a classic renal death. A blood test taken in Acapulco just before his doctors tried to get him to Houston to receive kidney dialysis showed high levels of the toxin, urea nitrogen. The actual blood level of codeine found in his blood at autopsy was high but not likely above his usual level considering his long-time tolerance and kidney failure. Murder by codeine administration cannot simply be proven based on his codeine blood level.

The use of codeine to blackmail Hughes into doing certain things is different. His medical history cannot precisely determine if he was ever threatened with codeine withholding unless he took certain actions. Unfortunately, history is filled with reports of persons who required opioids and who were blackmailed into doing something against their will by someone who controlled their supply of opioids. These ugly stories include women and even children forced into prostitution and young men forced into gangs and crime to get their heroin. Although there have been theories that codeine was withheld from HH to blackmail or force him to take actions he normally would not do, such as alter financial terms in employment contracts, there is no medical evidence or record to support this notion.

In 2007 I published a short article on the medical care of HH in "Practical Pain Management," a teaching journal for physicians of which I was the editor. Afterward I received a most revealing letter from Arelo Sederberg, who was the spokesman for the Hughes organization at the time of his death. The letter is reprinted here verbatim as it gives some insight into the thinking of executives inside the Hughes organization. It tends to negate any theories of intentional mistreatment of HH. The letter addressed to me and dated September 4, 2007 is quoted here as it helps "connect the dots" of HH's medical saga.

Dear Dr. Tennant,

I worked for Hughes from 1970 to 1978, so I was on board at the time of his death. In fact, I was the only spokesman then and throughout the estate mess. That's when all this stuff about his nuttiness came out, although there had been strong hints of it before. In all the years I saw him once and spoke to him twice. For the rest of my work – working with the press – I relied on Hughes aides and executives (who knew little more than I did, perhaps less). There was some fax corresponding too.

Sometimes I wonder if the Hughes aides (there were six) doctors (4) and executives (many, many, but only three counted at the end) weren't driven a little nutty through association. They were over cautious. I knew all these people well. They did, however, look upon me as a stranger since I had contact with the outside world. Interesting comment made by an aid (Johnny Holmes, who had been with Hughes for two decades) after the death of the Boss, "He was just an ordinary man. The press wants to make something out of it, but he was just an old man who died'.

Well, I be. A headliner for 50 years, an object of worldwide press interest (I received hundreds of calls from all over the world the day he died and continued to make news for two or three years after that) a record setter in aviation, an airplane designer without any formal schooling, a movie chieftain, a Las Vegas empire builder – just another guy? What it points out was that the closer you get to something the more ordinary it seems.

Best,

Arelo Sederberg

Arelo Sederberg reminds us about all of HH's contributions to society which had to be done by overcoming and coping with some horrific medical conditions.

The sex life of HH ceased about 10 years after his 1946 crash. His neurologic impairments and intractable pain were progressive after his plane crash primarily due to endocrine changes and neurologic damage. Impotence is routine in persons with IPS. TBI also causes hormone deficiencies. Multiple hormones including testosterone, the major sex driver, is diminished due to IPS and TBI as well as by opioids and other drugs needed to suppress pain.[34],[41] Today males and females with IPS and TBI can be tested for hormone deficiencies and given hormones to restore these deficiencies. Also, males today have access to such sex assisting drugs as Viagra® and even devices to assist with the erection ability. During HH's lifetime none of these advances were available. By the mid 1950's HH was about age 50 and his sex life had essentially come to an end. This fact probably played some part in his estrangement and divorce from Jean Peters. Most males and females with IPS lose all interest in sex unless they have access to today's hormone restorations. This clearly happened to HH.

On June 13, 2006, the front page of the Wall Street Journal published a story that seems highly improbable based on what we know about his medical conditions. A man by the name of Melvin Dummar claimed to have picked up HH in 1967 while he was found dazed face down on a desert road. Dummar produced a handwritten will which he claimed HH wrote and left him $156 million. This became known as the "Mormon Will" and it was declared fake in 1978 by a Las Vegas jury.

Amazingly, about 40 years later in 2006, a pilot by the name of Robert Derio came forward to support Dummar's long ago claim. He claimed that he periodically and secretly flew HH from Las Vegas northwest to the Cottontail Ranch Brothel in the year 1967. Mr. Derio claimed that HH had regular trysts with "Sunny," a redhead who had a diamond in an upper incisor. Mr. Derio claimed, "you couldn't see it unless she smiled broadly." He also claimed she was "class of the field." By Mr. Derio's account he fell asleep in the brothel's kitchen and woke up around 4:00 AM to find that HH had left the brothel. Derio claimed he flew back to Las Vegas by himself and was never again contacted by the Hughes entourage.

From a medical standpoint this story is unlikely in the sense that HH was 62 years old and certainly unable to have a normal sexual encounter due to his impotency and physical debilitation. He did not attempt much unassisted walking at this time of his life due to his injuries and neurologic impairments. His doctors had a difficult time getting him to walk much at all after about 1960, so it is unlikely he started to walk by himself down a desert road. Besides medical improbability the Hughes entourage claimed that he never left the Desert Inn between 1966 and 1970 when he departed for the Bahamas.

Debate has raged over the reason why HH became a recluse. There have been two popular theories. One is that his appearance had adversely changed, and he wanted people to remember him when he was young, handsome, and void of long hair and nails. The other is that his appearance in public would allow tax collectors and other parties to trace him. While there may be some validity to these two theories, his three medical conditions all tend to make one desire social isolation. For example, persons with OCD, TBI, and IPS tend to remain at home, have few close friends or acquaintances, and seldom leave home. Interestingly, today many persons with OCD, TBI, or IPS spend a great deal of time interacting with other people on social media who have the same disorder. It is not possible to point to a single reason for HH's reclusiveness, but the combination of his three major medical disorders certainly contributed to HH's penchant for reclusiveness and social isolation.

The popular conception of HH is that he was an addict. This belief is based on the definition of addict which tends to be different depending on whether or not you are a medical professional. To much of the public, anyone who takes a lot of opioids or other potentially abusable drug is an addict regardless of the reason the drug is taken. Medical professionals, in general, like to separate those persons who take opioids for a legitimate pain problem from those persons who take them for euphoria or other psychic need. The persons who do not have pain typically start one or more abusable drugs in their childhood or teenage years. HH did not start opioids until age 41 when he developed severe injuries and intractable pain after his 1946 air crash of the XF-11. He did not smoke or use marijuana and he rarely drank alcohol.

Most enlightened physicians like to call persons like HH who regularly take opioids strictly for pain suppression to be physically and therapeutically dependent rather than addicted. The term "pseudoaddict" has been used in recent years to separate pain patients who seek and need opioids from those who take opioids for psychologic, non-pain purposes. I have previously applied the term "pseudoaddict" to HH to educate medical personnel to not be prejudicial when a person asks for opioids. Does the person asking for opioids have a legitimate pain condition or are they just an addict looking for a psychic lift? Another popular myth is that he had poor medical care because he lived a secretive, reclusive life. This is simply not true. He recruited and hired excellent physicians and aides, some of whom had nursing-type backgrounds. He lived in luxury hotels with food prepared by the hotel dining service. Bedding, bathing, and toilet facilities were the finest. His physicians and aides tended to every medical issue, helped him eat, bathe, and use the toilet. In his last three years of life, he was bed-bound. Also, HH was somewhat savvy in that he knew to take a vitamin preparation. He even had a hobby he enjoyed – movie watching – which he was able to do almost daily until a few days before he died. Think of all the elderly people in nursing homes and assisted living facilities who would gladly move to the top floor of the Desert Inn!

Perhaps the biggest myth is that HH lived the last part of his life in depression, misery, and unhappiness. This was not the case. When HH moved into the top floor of the Desert Inn in 1966, at age 61, he obviously had decided to change his life, career, and set new goals for himself. He had survived a close brush with death after his XF-11 crash in 1946. He even told his physicians he "was prepared to die" during their successful and miraculous efforts to keep his heart and lungs pumping long enough for some healing to take place. In this author's long medical career, I have known and cared for numerous persons who felt the "kiss of death" and "heard the angels call" but managed to somehow survive a near-death experience. All felt blessed and came out of their ordeal with an altered view of life and some different goals. All, just like HH, also made good contributions to others after their near-death experience.

17. Why the Long Life?

"Hughes Lives to Age 70 Against Great Odds"

An old saying everyone knows is that cats have nine lives. The cats must have been buddies with HH! How he managed to live through four plane crashes is truly a miracle and a mystery. His survival in his last crash in 1946 was accomplished probably because his two doctors had extensive military and trauma experience. In fact, HH had many mysteries in his life, and he left one with us in his death. Why did he live so long? With his three major medical disorders, OCD, TBI, IPS, plus his genetic deafness, it is somewhat of a mystery as to why he lived to 70 years.

If the phenacetin in his main pain-relieving drug, codeine compound, as well as excessive Excedrin ® had not ruined his kidneys, he may have made it a few more years. His autopsy showed atherosclerosis in his coronary arteries and aorta, but not enough to likely do him in "real soon." In fact, his organs except his kidneys were in good enough condition to continue living at least a few more years. Even today with modern treatment of his three major conditions, most physicians would not expect him to live 70 years.

Is there a longevity lesson to be learned from HH? This question is explored in this chapter. First, we normally think that when someone lives longer than expected they have "good genes." His father and mother died at relatively young ages, however, so it certainly was not their genes if genes were a factor in his longevity. He amazingly survived four plane crashes and five episodes of concussion and unconsciousness. One must wonder if he just had a lot of luck or spiritual blessings from his God.

Despite popular labeling, HH was not a typical addict. He did not smoke and in the last two or three decades of his life he drank almost zero alcohol. Even though HH sometimes overused his two major medications, codeine and diazepam (Valium®), they likely also prolonged his life. They clearly helped control some of his IPS, OCD, and TBI symptoms in the last 10 to 11 years of his life. It is not possible to definitively answer this, but the non-codeine agents (aspirin, phenacetin, caffeine) in the compound were anti-inflammatory. His injections of codeine compound probably insured that these agents reached his brain and spinal canal and suppressed inflammation. To survive with IPS, one needs to get an inflammatory-suppressing agent into the brain. Diazepam may have not only helped his pain, but it may have provided some therapeutic suppression of his OCD and TBI symptoms.

His retreat into reclusiveness may have contributed to his longevity. Once he imbedded himself in luxury hotel suites which usually included a whole floor, he created several life-extending situations. First, he had the dollars to hire a stable of first-class aides and doctors to look after him. The activity logs kept between 1971 and 1973 showed that he slept, bathed on a regular basis, and ate healthy meals mainly of chicken and some carbohydrate-based desserts. Chicken is a dense protein that contains a great deal of tryptophan that makes serotonin which is vital for pain relief, depression, and helps with sleep. He received dressing changes for his skin ulcers (decubiti) and was given enemas when he needed them. He obviously enjoyed his one hobby which was watching movies. He had a high level of assisted living which was much better than one could usually obtain in the average assisted living quarters that are now in every American city. He stayed thin and his living quarters always had a lot of company around him. He was socially isolated from the outside world, but he had a lot of daily interactions with humans whom he liked.

Another possible longevity factor was that he took multivitamins. Dr. Thain thought HH's vitamin preparation was probably Theragram-M, but he was not positive about this. There is an undocumented report that claims he took a special-made vitamin-herbal preparation concocted by a Harvard nutritionist that contained several vitamins and herbs plus a high dose of selenium. This report was given to me several years ago by a salesperson for "Market America," a premier organization that sells many excellent nutritional products. Selenium is thought by many anti-aging physicians to be a life-extender.

Lastly, we know, from his physicians, a little about his mental state. All three of his physicians told me HH was eccentric and "neurotic" but neither depressed nor psychotic. He also had a sense of humor. He appeared to manage and enjoy his business activities right until the end. A telling event was that in 1966 at age 61 he decided to start a new career and lifestyle and reinvent Las Vegas. May we all have the motivation and health to make such a major life-move when we are in our 60's.

Good genes, protein diet, non-smoker, medical care, vitamins, thin, diazepam, codeine? We will never know exactly why he lived beyond what would be medically expected. It is clear, however, that he made some good decisions and beneficial moves to make it 70 years. He had to have that old intangible "will and want to live." There are writings that say HH must have died depressed, lonely, and addicted. Do not bet on it!

18. Summary

The medical saga of HH began at birth when he was born with hereditary obsessive-compulsive disorder (OCD) and partial deafness. He had an unusual upbringing as his mother had OCD. She was overly protective and afraid young Howard would contract polio or another infectious disease. He had several childhood medical symptoms that had no obvious cause and were apparently psychosomatic. At age 15 he even had an episode of paralysis with no medical basis. Besides exhibiting a variety of medical symptoms, his mechanical and engineering genius emerged. Before age 15 he had developed a ham radio, built a motorized bicycle, and tore down and rebuilt a Stutz Bearcat automobile.

Between the ages of 17 and 19 his mother and father died. The courts in Houston, Texas declared him an emancipated minor and he inherited 75% of the Hughes Tool Company which was worth millions. HH's father had a patent on a drill bit that would cut through packed sand and rock to extract oil and gas, which generated millions of dollars. HH used this money to build his film, aviation, and entertainment enterprises. At age 20 in 1925 he married Ella Rice and moved to Los Angeles to enter the new silent film industry in which his uncle Rupert was a top producer. Before the age of 21 he had hired Noah Dietrich to oversee his new Hollywood film operation while he ran the tool company. Within only three years, he and Dietrich made some popular and profitable silent films. HH chose to direct and fly a plane in the movie

"Hell's Angels." Against the advice of expert pilots, HH flew a scout plane too close to the ground and he crashed. He was knocked unconscious and hospitalized. This was the first of his four plane crashes and numerous accidents resulting in traumatic brain injury (TBI). After the "Hell's Angels" air crash and brain injury, his symptoms of OCD started to be more severe and regular. His major symptoms were germaphobia, repetitious behaviors, and perfectionistic desires. TBI symptoms also emerged as evidenced by memory lapses and poor decision making.

Between 1928 and 1951 HH had at least a dozen episodes of bodily trauma of which five resulted in concussions and coma. Three automobile accidents caused his head to hit the windshield which required sutures to close face and scalp lacerations. He had physical altercations with Ava Gardner, and two men whose wife or ex-wife he was dating.

The event that drastically changed his life and health occurred in 1946 when he crashed an experimental, Army reconnaissance plane, the XF-11. He miraculously lived thanks to the expertise of two physicians with war-time experiences, Drs. Lawrence Chaffin, and Vernon Mason. He suffered so many burns, trauma, and tissue damage that he later developed a condition now referred to as Intractable Pain Syndrome (IPS). This relatively rare disorder is constant (24/7) incurable pain that has cardiovascular and endocrine complications. By age 50 his health began to deteriorate, and he dropped out of public life to live a reclusive and secretive existence. Dr. Verne Mason started HH on the mild opioid, codeine, which he took almost daily, at moderately high dosages, over a period of 30 years between 1946 and 1976 until he died at age 70. The cause was a result of kidney failure due to phenacetin which was a component in codeine compound plus excessive Excedrin®. When diazepam (Valium®) came on the commercial market in 1963, he was started on it and it appeared to lessen his OCD/TBI symptoms enough to help him function and make his move and transition to Las Vegas. He changed his life and career in 1966 at age 61 when he moved into the top floor of the Desert Inn in Las Vegas. He had visions to change Vegas from a shoddy gambling town to an entertainment and scientific mecca. Today's Las Vegas owes a lot to his efforts. In 1970 he left Las Vegas to live out his life in luxury hotels in various countries. He accepted his plight and carried on business from his hotel right up until a few days before his death. He died on April 5, 1976 in route to Methodist Hospital in Houston from Acapulco, Mexico.

HH suffered from three major medical conditions: OCD, TBI, and IPS. In his lifetime these conditions were hardly recognized or understood. If the treatments used today had been available, the entire persona and saga of HH would undoubtedly be quite different. Amazingly he lived 70 years with his medical conditions. A good part of his survival was obviously his intellect and will to live. Overlooked is that he had the foresight and money to hire excellent doctors and aides and lived in luxury hotels that had first class dietary and housekeeping services.

The medical saga of HH is clearly one of a kind. He was the richest man in the world during his life and coped with OCD, TBI, IPS, and deafness. He overcame them enough to give society many enduring contributions. He contributed millions to his Howard Hughes Medical Institute which until this day sponsors medical research. His own medical saga may, however, provide more knowledge, education, and benefits over time to humankind than will his institute.

HE CAME

HE SAW

HE CONQUERED

This message was on a red, white, and blue ribbon attached to a five-foot high, airplane shaped arrangement of pompoms sent to his burial service from an anonymous Southern California Fitness Club.

SPECIAL NOTE: I came, I saw, I conquered is a Latin phrase that Julius Caesar wrote in a letter to the Roman Senate around 47 BC, after he had a swift, conclusive victory over Pharnaces II of Pontus, the King of the Mediterranean Territory known as Cimmerian Bosporus.

19. Selected Bibliography

1.Bartlett DL, Steele JB. Empire: The Life, Legend, and Madness of Howard Hughes. WW Norton & Co., New York, 1979.

2.Baxter C, Haworth J. Howard Hughes, His Other Empire and His Man. Vantage Press, 1996.

3.Breo D. Howard Hughes in Extra Care. American Medical Association, Chicago, Ill,1986.

4.Brown PH, Broeski F. Howard Hughes: The Untold Story. Penguin Books USA, INC. New York, 1996.

5.Davenport E, Eddy P, Hurwitz M. The Hughes Papers. Ballantine Books, New York, NY 1976.

6.Dietrich N, Thomas B. Howard: The Amazing Mr. Hughes. Fawcett Publication Inc., Greenwich, Conn, 1972,1976; pp304-305.

7.Drosnin M. Citizen Hughes. Holt, Fineham and Winston. New York, 1985.

8.Hack R. Hughes: The Private Diaries, Memos, and Letters. New Millenium Press, Beverly Hills, CA, 2001.

9.Longworth K. Seduction, Sex, Lies, and Stardom in Howard Hughes Hollywood. Custom House, 2018.

10.Maheau R, Hack R. Next to Hughes. Harper Collins Publishers, New York, NY, 1992.

11.Phelan J. Howard Hughes: The Hidden Years. Warner Books, New York, NY, 1976.

SPECIAL NOTE: Many of the vignettes, stories, and events that are in this book have been excerpted from one or more of the books in this bibliography.

20. Medical References

1. Apkarian AV, Sosa Y, Sont S, et al. Chronic back pain is associated with decreased prefrontal and thalamic gray matter density. J Neurosci 2004;24(46):10410-10415.

2. Austin PJ, Moaleno-Taylor G. The neuro-immune balance in neuropathic pain: involvement of inflammatory immune cells, immune-like glial cells and cytokines. J Neuroimmunol 2010;229:26-50.
3. Berrios GE. Obsessive compulsive disorder: its conceptual history in France during the 19th century. Comp Psych 1989;30(4):283-295.
4. Burns E, Kakara R. Deaths from falls among persons aged >65 years-United States, 2007-2016. MMWR Morb Mortal Wkly 2018;67:509-514.

5. Cauda F, Palermo S, Costa T, et al. Gray matter alterations in chronic pain: a network-oriented-meta-analytic approach. Neuroimage Clin 2014;4(Apr 16):676-688.

6. Caufield DA, Sorris J, Berk. Nutraceuticals in the treatment of obsessive-compulsive disorder (OCD): a review of mechanistic and clinical evidence. 2011;35(4):887-895.
7. Coutinho ES, Block KV, Coeli CM. One-year mortality among elderly people after hospitalization due to fall-related fractures: comparison with a control group of matched elderly. CAD Saude Publica 2012;28(4):81-805.

8. Daly RM. Exercise and nutritional approaches to prevent frail bones, falls, and fractures: an update. Climacteric 2017;20(2):119-24.
9. Davidson J, Bjorgvinsson T. Current and potential pharmacological treatments for obsessive-compulsive disorder. Expert Opinion on Investigational Drugs 2003;12(6):993-1001.
10. Dittman M. Hughes germ phobia revealed in psychological autopsy. Amer Psy Ass 2005;36(7):102.
11. Eddy KT, Dutra L, Bradley, et al. A multidimensional meta-analysis of psychotherapy and pharmacotherapy for obsessive-compulsive disorder. Clin Psychol Rev 2004;24(8):1011-1030.
12. Etsy ML, Shifflett CM. Head injuries in history in Conquering Concussion, Round Earth Publishing, Sewickly, PA 2014,pp1-19.
13. Fenske JN, Schwenk TL. Obsessive-compulsive disorder: diagnosis and management. Amer Fam Phys 2009;80(3):239-245.
14. Fine PG. Long-term consequences of chronic pain: mounting evidence for pain as a neurologic disease and parallels with other chronic disease states. Pain Med 2011;12(1):996-1004.
15. Gdolevich M, Cohen D, Yosef D, et al. Morbidity and mortality after hip fracture: the impact of operative delay. Arch Orthop Trauma Surg 2004;124:334-340.
16. Glynn CJ, Lloyd JW. Biochemical changes associated with intractable pain. Br Med J 1978;1:280-281.
17. Goodman WK, Grice DE, Lapidus KA, et al. Obsessive-compulsive disorder. Psych Clinic No Amer 2014;37(3):257-267.
18. Haring RS, Narang K, Canner JK, et al. Traumatic brain injury in the elderly: morbidity and mortality trends and risk factors. J Surg Res 2015;195(1):1-9.
19. Hoge CW, Goldberg HM, Castro CA. Care of war veterans with mild traumatic brain injury. N Engl J Med 2009;360(16):1588-1591.
20. Javidi E, Magnus T. Autoimmunity after ischemic stroke and brain injury. Fron in Immun 2019;10:1-12.

21. Kallia P, Walling A. Obsessive-compulsive disorders in Current Therapy 2020, pp796-799.
22. Koran LM. Obsessive-compulsive disorder: an update for the clinician. Focus 2007;(5):3.
23. Kremer M, Yalcin L, Goumun Y, et al. A dual-adrenergic mechanism for the relief of neuropathic allodynia by the antidepressant drugs duloxetine and amitriptyline. J Neurosci 2018;38:9934-9954.
24. Latremoliere A, Woolf CJ. Central sensitization: a generator of pain hypersensitivity by central neural plasticity. J Pain 2009;10:895-926.
25. Maroon JC, Field M, Lovell M, et al. The evaluation of athletes with cerebral concussion. Clin Neurosurg 2002;49:319-332/
26. Marchi N, Bozarian JJ, Puvenna V, et al. Consequences of repeated blood brain disruption in football players. PLOS ONE 2013;8(3):e56805.
27. Martikaineh K, et al. Chronic pain is associated with alterations in dopamine neurotransmission in the ventral striatum. J Neurosci 2015;35:9957-9965.
28. May A, Boorsok D, Becerra L. Chronic pain may change the structure of the brain. Pain 2008; 137(1):7–15. 28.
29. McKee AC, Cantu RC, Nowinski CJ, et al. Chronic traumatic encephalopathy in athletes: progressive tauopathy after resitive head injury. J Neuropath Exp Neurol 2009;68(7):709-735.
30. Mika J, Zychowska M, Popiolek-Barczy K, et al. Importance of glial activation in neuropathic pain. Eur J Pharmacol 2013;716:106-119.
31. Millon MJ. Descending control of pain. Prog Neurobiol 2002;66:355-474.
32. Moltner A, Holz R, Strian F. Heart rate changes as an autonomic component of the pain response. Pain 1990;43(1):81-89.
33. Raffaeli W, Arando E. Pain as a disease: an overview. J Pain Res 2017;10:2003-2008.
34. Schneider HJ, Kreitschmann-Andermahr I, Ghigo E, et al. Hypothalmopituitary dysfunction following traumatic brain

injury and aneurysmal subarachnoid hemorrhage: a systematic review. J Amer Med Assoc 2007;298(12):1429-1438.
35. Schnell S, Friedman SM, Mendelson DA, et al. The 1-year mortality of patients treated in a hip fracture program for elders. Geriatric Orthop Surg & Rehab 2010;1:6-14.
36. Shenkin HA. Effect of pain on diurnal pattern of plasma corticoid levels. Neurology 1964;14:1112-1115.
37. Stern RA, Riley DO, Daneshuar DH, et al. Long-term consequences of repetitive brain trauma: chronic traumatic encephalopathy. PMR 2011;3:S460-S467.
38. ubramaneau M, Soh P, Vaingankar JA et al. Quality of life in obsessive-compulsive disorder: impact of the disorder and of treatment. CNS Drugs 2013;27(5):367-383.
39. Tennant F, Hermann L. Intractable or chronic pain: there is a difference. West J Med 2000;173:306.
40. Tennant F. The physiologic effects of pain on the endocrine system. Pain Ther 2013;2:75.86.
41. Tennant F. Hormone abnormalities in severe, chronic pain patients who fail standard treatment. Postgrad Med 2015;127(1):1-4.
42. Tracey I, Bushnell MC. How neuroimaging studies have challenged us to rethink: is chronic pain a disease? J Pain 2009;10(11):1113–1120.
43. Walsh Js. Normal bone physiology, remodeling, and its hormonal regulation. Surgery 2015;33(1):1-6.
44. Wood T, Murganti-Kossman MC. The role of markers of inflammation in traumatic brain injury. Fron in Neurol 2013;4:1-12.
45. Wu K, Hanna GL, Rosenburg DR, et al. The role of glutamate signaling in the pathogenesis and treatment of obsessive-compulsive disorder. Pharm Biochem & Behav 2012;100(4):726-735.

21. Chronology of Medically Related Events

AGE	DATE	EVENT
0	Dec. 24, 1905	Born in Humble, Texas with hereditary obsessive-compulsive disorder and partial deafness. Named Howard Robard Hughes, Jr.
1	Oct. 7, 1906	Certificate of Baptism, St. John's Episcopal Church, Keokuk, Iowa.
3	1908	Hughes father files for patent on revolutionary oil drilling bit.
11	1916	Built a ham-radio and became licensed as an operator.
12	1917	Build a motorized bicycle with parts from his father's steam engine.
14	1919	Took first flying lesson.
15	1920	Developed paralysis of legs with no known cause. Spontaneously resolved.
16-19	1921-24	Attended various schools including Fessenden School in Massachusetts, Caltech, and Rice University.
17	1922	Mother, Allene Hughes, died of an ectopic pregnancy
19	1924	Father Howard Hughes, Sr. died of heart attack. HH declared an emancipated minor and inherited 75% of the Hughes estate.

20	June 1, 1925	Marries Ella Botts Rice and moves to Los Angeles.
20	Nov.1925	Hires Noah Dietrich as chief executive of his operations.
21	1926	Produces his first film "Swell Hogan" which was never shown.
22	1927	Begins producing Hell's Angels.
23	January 29, 1928	Plane crash filming "Hell's Angels." Unconscious. Hospitalized. Met Dr. Vernon Mason.
24	June 1, 1929	Developed spinal meningitis. Comatose. Recovered.
24	Dec. 9, 1929	Divorces Ella Botts Rice.
26	1931	Contracted syphilis. Treated with mercury and arsenic with apparent recovery.
27	1932	Automobile accident. Hit windshield. Lacerations on tip of his head sutured by Dr. Lawrence Chaffin.
30	1935	Crash landed his H-1 airplane in a beet field apparently because he ran out of gas.
31	July 11, 1936	Hughes struck and killed a pedestrian named Gabriel S. Meyer. There were questions of his sobriety, but he was not charged with negligent homicide.
33	1938	Dr. Vern Mason and Dr. Norman Crane, both internists, shared offices in the Pacific Mutual Building in Los Angeles. Mason was HH's personal physician but introduced him to Dr. Norman Crane.
35	1940	Car crash threw him head-first through a windshield. Required hospitalization.

38	1943	Ava Gardner hits him with a bronze bell smashing him between the temple and cheekbone. Knocked out two teeth and gave him a scalp gash that required 22 stitches. Was unconscious.
39	May 17, 1943	Plane crash in Sikorskys-43 Amphibian Aircraft at Lake Mead. Propeller blade came through the passenger compartment. Two persons killed. Hughes had large gash on top of his head closed with clips and he suffered a concussion.
39	Fall/1944	Suffers what was called a nervous breakdown while making Hercules Flying Boat (Spruce Goose).
41	1944	Automobile accident with lacerations on the right side of his face. Required sutures by Dr. Lawrence Chaffin.
41	July 7, 1946	XF-11 reconnaissance plane crashes in Culver City, CA. Severe injuries. Grows mustache to hide scars on his upper lip. Codeine prescribed for pain by Dr. Vernon Mason, after Hughes leaves hospital on August 11, 1946.
42	April 5,1947	Successfully test flies second FX-11 at Culver City.
42	August 6-10, 1947	Testifies before Senate War Investigating Committee probing his work as a defense contractor. Very articulate and persuasive.
42	Oct 1947	Frank William (Bill) Gay goes to work at Romain Street, Los Angeles headquarters.
42	1947-48	Gains control of RKO Production Company (films, radio stations, theaters). Forms Hughes Helicopters, and focusses on being a major defense contractor.
42	Nov., 1947	Test flew Hercules (Spruce Goose) at Long Beach for one mile.

43	May 10, 1948	Acquires control of RKO Production Studios.
44	1949	Apparent phony marriage to Terry Moore while on a boat. No trace of marriage certificate.
46	1951	Glenn Davis, a former football star, became engaged to Terry Moore. Hughes sent Terry's engagement ring to Davis and he attacked Hughes re-breaking his ribs and chin.
48	1953	Forms Howard Hughes Medical Institute and gives all his Hughes Aircraft stock to the Institute. Dr. Vernon Mason heads medical advisory board.
48	Dec. 17, 1953	Howard Hughes Medical Institute incorporated in Delaware.
49	1954	Sells RKO companies at a profit of $25 million.
50	Feb. 11, 1953	Takes last pilots' test in Miami, Florida.
52	Jan. 12, 1957	Marries Jean Peters in Tonopah, Nevada.
52	May 12, 1957	Fires Noah Dietrich.
53	1958	Has what is called a "nervous breakdown." Teenage consort claims HH to be impotent.
52-55	1956-60	Rift with top aide, Noah Dietrich, who reportedly tried to claim that Hughes was mentally incompetent. Aides report that Hughes became quite reclusive with poor hygiene and compulsive movie watching. Forced out of TWA management.
56	Dec. 1, 1961	Dr. Norman Crane becomes HH's personal physician after retirement of Dr. Vern Mason. Begins prescribing codeine to HH.
57	1962-64	Acquired control of Boston-based Northeast

		Airlines. Sold it in 1964. Dr. Crane starts diazepam (Valium®) which helps control his OCD/TBI symptoms.
61	July 17, 1966	Went to Boston to ostensibly seek medical care. No documentation that this occurred. Stayed at Ritz-Carlton Hotel.
61	Nov.24, 1966	Hughes begins moving into Desert Inn, sets up business and purchases multiple hotel-casinos and local television stations between 1966-68.
61	Nov. 27, 1966	Arrives in Las Vegas by train from Boston taking over top floor of the Desert Inn.
63	1968	Hughes Tool Company purchases North Las Vegas air Terminal.
63	1968-69	Pathologist Homer Clark, MD did laboratory work on HH and selected a blood donor.
65	1970	Acquired San Francisco-based Air West and renamed it Hughes Air west
65	Nov. 26, 1970	Left Las Vegas for Bahamas. Did not return to USA until death.
65	1970	Fires Robert Maheu as chief of operations.
65	1970	Required a pint of blood for anemia. Taken to Nassau, Bahamas from Salt Lake City by hematologist, Homer Clark, MD.
66	Feb.,1971	Had pressure sore on his buttocks and over his left scapula. There were sinus tracts under the scapula sores. Dr. Chaffin summoned to treat them.
66	1971	Divorce from Jean Peters. Lifetime alimony payment of $70,000 a year. She refused all media requests. Had not seen Hughes for several years.
67	March 14, 1972	Departed Managua, Nicaragua and arrived at Bayshore Inn Hotel in Vancouver, Canada.

67	Aug. 1972	Dr. Wilbur Thain makes 1st visit to HH. Location - Vancouver, British Columbia.
67	Aug. 29, 1972	Departed Vancouver for the Intercontinental Hotel in Nicaragua.
67	January 7, 1972	Telephone interview from Bahamas with newsmen in Los Angeles to refute Clifford Irvine book.
67	May 12, 1973	Personally flew 1st of 4 successful flights out of London in a new Hawker-Siddeley twin engine turboprop. Flew undressed from waist down.
67	May 1973	Dr. Thain discussed vitamin/mineral preparation with HH.
67	July 13, 1973	Dr. Lawrence Chaffin summoned to assist with decubiti, imbedded needles, and rectal prolapse. Becomes regular attending physician.
67	August 9, 1973	Fell and fractured hip in London. Pinned in London Hospital. Never walked afterward.
67	1973	Wilbur Thain, MD starts attending HH in London and named head physician.
67	Dec. 1973	HH moved from London to Xanadu Hotel in Freeport, Bahamas.
68	April 26, 1974	Dr. Crane informs Dr. Thain that he will no longer prescribe codeine and Valium® to HH. Dr. Thain takes over as head physician.
68	Aug. 3, 1974	Seven-hour meeting with HH and Drs. Thain and Crane. Purpose: put HH on forced withdrawal program to be off codeine and Valium® by Dec. 24, 1974.
69	1975	Dr. Chaffin removed a broken needle from the back of HH's left upper arm. Dr. Chaffin ordered a portable x-ray to aid in removing any broken fragments of the needles, but HH never allowed it to be used. At least on broken-off

		needle worked its way out without treatment.
69-70	Nov. 1974 to death April 1976	Dr. Thain gives HH 48 codeine and 6 Valium® a week. HH escalates Excedrin® use to 12 to 20 tablets a day.
70	Feb., 1976	HH moved from Freeport to Acapulco, Mexico.
70	April 5, 1976 1:27 PM	Died in route from Acapulco to Houston. Press release by Methodist Hospital gave cause of death to be renal failure.
70	April 6, 1976	Permission for autopsy given by William R. Lummis on behalf of his mother Mrs. F.R. Lummis, Sr., next of kin. Autopsy performed between 1:30 and 3:10 PM.
70	April 7, 1976	Buried in the family plot at the Glenwood Cemetery in Houston.
70	April 10, 1976	Toxicology report reveals codeine in body fluids. Dr. Jack Titus attends the annual seminar of the Houston Society of Clinical Pathologists and refuses requests for additional information about HH and his autopsy.

APPENDIX

*All documents in the appendix are verbatim duplicates of the original documents. All were public evidence in the federal trial, United States versus Wilbur Thain, MD.

MEDICAL REVIEW OF HOWARD R. HUGHES

September 10, 1978

By

Forest S. Tennant, Jr., M.D., Dr. P.H.
Community Health Projects, Inc.
336½ South Glendora Avenue
West Covina, California 91790
(213) 919-5807

And

Assistant Professor
Division of Epidemiology
UCLA School of Public Health
UCLA Center for Health Services
Los Angeles, California 900024

Prepared For:

United States Government

INDEX F0R CASE-REVIEW OF HOWARD R. HUGHES (HRH)

I. Introduction

II. Review Materials, Findings, and Interpretation
  A. Letter from Gary Elliott to Forest Tennant, M.D.
    1. Findings
    2. Calculation to determine if enough codeine prescribed to maintain addiction
    3. Interpretation
  B. Death Certificate
  C. Fingerprints
  D. Birth Certificate
  E. Statements of Identification by Physicians
  F. Authorization for Autopsy
  G. Toxicologic Examination
    1. Findings
    2. Calculation to determine dose of codeine taken by HRH just before death
    3. Interpretation
  H. Laboratory Studies
    1. Findings
    2. Interpretation
  I. Autopsy Report
    1. General appearance at death
    2. Major diagnoses
  J. X-ray of Arms
  K. Memorandum from HRH to Staff regarding Medical Prescriptions, Date: October 2, 1958
  L. Log of HRH's Activities kept by Aides between Oct. 31, 1971, and July 1, 1973

1. Content
2. Major activities
3. Medical notes

M. Personal Communication with Special Agent, Gary Elliott, regarding HRH's Medical and Drug HistoryChronological Health History

I. Legal Aspects of Case

a. Facts Bearing on Case

II. References

III. INTRODUCTION

In June, 1978, I was requested by Special Agent, Gary Elliott, and Assistant U.S. Attorney, Max Wheeler, to be a United States Government consultant involving alleged illegal and inappropriate prescribing and administrating of narcotics by Wilbur S. Thain, M.D., for the deceased, Howard R. Hughes (HRH). The essence of this report and any public testimony or information that I may give is based on my review of materials and information supplied to me by Mr. Elliott and my knowledge of the various aspects of narcotic use and abuse.

This short report contains some scientific, medical, and legal references to help substantiate the opinions given here.

I. REVIEW MATERIALS, FINDINGS, AND INTERPRETATION

Listed here are the review materials made available to me. Of considerable medical and legal importance is that HRH's physicians kept no medical records on HRH.

B. <u>Letter from Gary Elliott to Forest Tennant, M.D.</u>

1. <u>Findings</u>

Codeine Phosphate, Empirin-Codeine®, ad Valium® were supplied to HRH between August, 1974, and April, 1976. Between August 6, 1974, and December 13, 1975, Dr. Wilbur Thain ordered and received 5,500 dosage units of Codeine Phosphate. (Were 60 mg. or 1 gr. Injectable tablets), which was the maximal amount that HRH could have consumed between August 1974 and April 7, 1976 (death).

2. Calculation to Determine if Enough Codeine Prescribed to Maintain Addiction

Given here is a simple mathematic calculation to determine if HRH was prescribed enough codeine Phosphate between August 6, 1974, and December 13, 1975, to be addicted assuming every dose was taken which was apparently not the case. Total codeine dose of 5500 grains = 9.14 grains (548 mg) per day, 602 days between 8/6/74 and 12/13/75.

3. Interpretation

The amount of Codeine Phosphate prescribed by Dr. W. Thain to HRH during this period is more than enough to maintain physical addiction.[1-7] A daily codeine dose of 500 to 800 mg. is similar to the dosages consumed by codeine addicts who seek treatment.[8] The doses of codeine prescribed to and consumed by JRJ could only be done by a person who had consumed codeine on a chronic basis and developed tolerance to it. Here are general guidelines concerning codeine:

a. Usual prescribed pain-relieving dose, 30-60 mg, every 4-6 hours[3,6]
b. Toxic dose in non-tolerant person, over 200-300 mg, in single dose[3,7]
c. Death dose in non-tolerant person, over 500-800 mg, in single dose[7]

C. Death Certificate

Death Date April 7, 1976 – Age 70
Immediate Cause: Chronic Renal Failure doe to Chronic Interstitial Nephritis with Papillary Necrosis

D. Fingerprints of HRH – no pertinent information to Case-Review

E. Birth Certificate of HRH – Born December 24, 1905

F. Statements of Identification by Wilbur S. Thain, M.D., Lawrence Chaffin, M.D., and John Morrison Holmes. No significant information regards Case-Review.

G. Authorization for Autopsy by Annette G. Lummis (aunt of HRH), by William R. Lummis (son of Annette G. Lummis). No significant information regards Case-Review.

H. Toxicologic Examination of HRH at Death

Blood, urine, and other body fluids were taken from HRH at the time of autopsy.

1. Findings

Alcohol = Negative (Cerebrospinal fluid)
Barbiturates = Negative (Blood)
Acetylsalicylic Acid = Negative (Blood)
Drug Screen = Negative (Blood, Urine, Liver, and Stomach contents)
Phenacetin = Negative (Blood, Urine, Liver, and Stomach contents)
Narcotics: 0.196 mg. % Codeine (Blood)
4.8 mg. % Codeine (Bile)
6.6 mg. Codeine (Urine)
0.7 mg. % Codeine (Liver)
2.2 mg. Codeine (Stomach contents)

2. Calculation to determine dose of codeine taken by HRH just before death

a. 42 Kilograms (Weight of HRH at death) x.09 (Blood volume is 8.5-9.0% of body weight) 3.78 Liters of 3780 ml.
b. .196 mg. Codeine in HRH blood= x Approx. amount of codeine 100 ml. 3780 ml. in blood volume x (Approximate minimal amount) = 7.41 mg. Minimal amount of Codeine consumed in 4-6 hours before death.

3. Interpretation

The amount of codeine found in the blood of JRJ at death is very compatible with tolerance and addiction to codeine. It also correlates reasonably well with known amounts prescribed to him. Codeine is one of the fastest acting and most rapidly metabolized narcotics, and it remains in the blood stream for only 4 to 6 hours after consumption. Since higher levels of codeine were found in the bile and urine than in the blood,[2,5,7] it is likely that HRH was tolerant to codeine, a blood level many times higher than the level found here would be required to produce death.

I. Laboratory Studies on HRH

Blood was drawn in Acapulco about 48 hours before death when HRH's aides and physicians realized that he was seriously ill. This blood was apparently available for testing at Methodist Hospital in Houston.

1. Findings		
	Blood Taken 2 days Before Death	Blood Taken Immediately After Death
Blood Urea Nitrogen (Normal 8-24 mg/dl)	47 mg dl	60mg/dl
Creatinine (Normal .5-1.5 mg/dl)	1.4 mg dl	20 mg/dl

2. Interpretation
The pertinent blood studies indicate renal failure (e.g., "uremic poisoning"), and they are compatible with finding that there was atrophic kidneys due to long-term phenacetine abuse.

J. Autopsy Report from Methodist Hospital, Houston, Texas, April, 1976

1. General Appearance at Death
    a. Weight – 42 kilograms (87 pounds)
    b. Height – 185 cm. (72.7 inches)
    c. Elderly appearance
    d. Gray hair, thinned and gray beard
    e. Small bed sores

2. Major Diagnoses
    a. Granular atrophy of kidneys with necrosis of most renal papillae due to phenacetin abuse (found in Empirin-Codeine®)
    b. Aden fibromatoses Hyperplasia of prostate with partial urethral obstruction
    c. Moderate urethral stricture
    d. Renal failure
    e. Emaciation and dehydration*

*May have been terminal event since kidneys weighed 200 gms and may have been good enough to survive longer.

3. Accessory Diagnoses
    a. Fibrotic apical scars both lungs and old, fibrotic left pleural adhesions (history of old left thoracic injury)
    b. Metallic pin left hip from repair of prior fracture

c. Contusion of left shoulder
d. Chronic peptic gastric ulcer
e. Single focus of 60% atherosclerotic narrowing of mid left descending coronary artery
f. Focal complex atherosclerotic lesions of aorta
g. Adenoma (2 cm) right lobe of thyroid
h. Single left vertebral artery
i. Moderate dilation occipital portions of lateral cerebral ventricles
j. Ulcerated nodule of scalp (cystic adenocarcinoma)
k. Multiple needle punctures and ecchymoses forearm – fresh
l. Moderate contractures (15-20^0 flexion) of both knees (history of not walking for about 3 years since fracture of hip)
m. Osteoporosis
n. Diverticulosis of colon
o. Dental caries – severe – evidence of neglect

K. X-Ray of Arms of HRH

A remarkable x-ray of HRH's arms reveal four broken, imbedded needle points (about ½ inch each) in the subcutaneous tissues of the right arm. One needle point is imbedded in the left arm. Superficial veins are calcified as a result of venous infections, inflammation, and/or intravenous injection of insoluble materials. This is frequently found with the injection of non-narcotic compounds like those found in Empirin®.[9-11]

L. Memorandum from HRH to Staff regarding Medical Prescriptions, Date: October 2, 1958

This memoranda gives very detailed instructions to staff on how to secure and process prescriptions including triplicate (narcotic) prescriptions. These instructions do not impress me as being flexible enough to obtain sufficient quantities of narcotics (e.g. codeine or other) to be addicted, although the memorandum displays a knowledge of procedures to obtain narcotics. They do appear to be compatible with intermittent misuse, over-medication, and abuse of drugs.

M. Log of HRH's Activities kept by Aides between Oct. 31, 1971, and July 1, 1973

1. Content

This detailed log was kept by HRH's aides and records the specific time of each day that HRH engaged in various activities, including the following:

a. Used bathroom
b. Ate
c. Watched films or television
d. Sat in chair reading
e. Took drugs and type of drug
f. Transacted business
g. Left hotel

2. Major Activities and Drug Use

Several points relevant to the medical and drug history of HRH are found in this log. These points are summarized:

a. Diet consisted mostly of chicken, but HRH ate regularly.
b. HRH was apparently very constipated since he took as many as 20-25 laxative (Surfax®) capsules in one dose.
c. Was regular user of diazepam (Valium®), 10 mg., and HRH's aides usually referred to them in the log as BB's ("Blue Bomber" since they are a blue tablet). HRH would often consume as many as 9 (90 mg.) Valium® which indicates considerable tolerance, long-term previous consumption, and possibly physical addiction.
d. Codeine was consumed on an irregular basis, but in very large doses. It was usually consumed as Empirin #4 (60 mg. of codeine with aspirin 227 mg.; phenacetin 162 mg.; and caffeine 32 mg.). On many days during this period he consumed, in one dose, 10 or 12 Empirin® which is 600 to 720 mg. One notation indicates he consumed 25 Empirin (1500 mg.) in one dose. These doses indicate tremendous tolerance and considerable previous consumption of narcotics since single doses of about 800 mg. are often fatal in the normal human. It is not possible to determine form this log if HRH was physically addicted to codeine since most days during this period do not indicate codeine use.
e. Beginning on June 14, 1972, there are notations that HRH engaged in the "Big E." This usually occurred in the bathroom which suggests that the "big E" was an enema.
f. The log indicates that HRH could mentally function well at least intermittently during this period of time. HRH transacted some business,

including stock sales, leases, and tax decisions. He met with President Somoza of Nicaragua on March 13, 1972.

On at least one occasion he left his hotel to fly a plane. He frequently read newspapers. The log also recounts the famous telephone interview on January 7, 1972, regarding the infamous and fraudulent Clifford Irving biography and later signings with McGraw-Hill and affidavits for the New York Supreme Court. He made several trips and stayed in numerous locations, including Managua, Miami, Vancouver, and England.

3. Medical Notes	
Note	My Interpretation
a. Aides changed bandages on 2 occasions, and at least 2 falls, including 1 from toilet stool.	Possible skin infections at site of injections and /or from Falls. Occasional falls would be expected with his high dose of sedatives and narcotics.
b. Same spoon always used for Medicine.	No record of liquid medication, so I assume this spoon was used to dissolve codeine in water for self-administration.
c. Complained of frequent chilliness and sensitiveness temperature change.	Chills are frequent when blood levels of a narcotic such as codeine drop. Could also possibly be related to progressive renal failure (e.g., "uremic poisoning") or individual trait.
d. Dr. Clark visited only one time. No other recorded physician visits, lab tests, or medical records. No mention of how medications obtained.	Highly unusual to have so much prescription medication and only one physician visit.
e. Hair, beard, nails occasionally trimmed by aides. No mention of tooth brushing.	Partially explained poor dental condition noted at death.
f. Complained of "illness" only one time. No recorded complaints of pain.	Cause unknown. Possibly narcotic withdrawal, minor infection, or progression of uremia.
g. Concealment of medication habit indicated only one time when HRH instructed	May have been effort to conceal intravenous drug use, other medication habit, or even unrelated

	aides not to empty trash in bathroom until permission was given, No mention of syringes.	to drugs.
h.	Unusual obsessions and habits only indicated in requests for Kleenexes and special preparation of bedding. No hallucinations of delusions.	Habits appeared peculiar or "eccentric" but no real evidence of a psychotic or severe mental disorder.

N. Personal Communication with Special Agent, Gary Elliott, regarding HRH's Medical and Drug History

Special Agent, Gary Elliott, diligently obtained considerable information regarding pertinent facts concerning the medical and drug history about HRH. He obtained this additional information from interviews with:

HRH's physicians
HRH's aides

Pertinent points are:

1. HRH was in a widely-publicized plane crash in 1946. He was administered large amounts of morphine* while in the hospital, but it is unknown if he became addicted.
2. HRH began using Empirin®-codeine after leaving the hospital, but the precise amounts and frequency of use are unknown. It is unknown if HRH was ever addicted to codeine prior to 1970's.
3. HRH sustained a fall in London in 1973 (Log's last date is 7/1/73) which fractured his hip and required a metal pin for repair. HRH never walked again.

*Morphine is a narcotic pain reliever very closely related to codeine. When taken internally, codeine partially converts to morphine.

II. Chronological Health History

Based on review of the facts available to me, I summarize HRH's health and drug history as follows:

Date	**Age in Years**	**Event**
1946	41	Plane accident with severe injuries. Exposed to high doses of the narcotic, morphine.
1947-1958	42-53	Intermittent overuse of Empirin® (codeine, aspirin, phenacetin, caffeine) and possibly other drugs.
1958	53	HRH gives detailed instructions to staff to insure that prescription drugs are available in quantities large enough to misuse, over-medicate, and abuse. Addiction not evident.
1958-1971	53-66	Increasing misuse and abuse of prescription medications, particularly Empirin®, medications. Health and work function not significantly impaired. Intermittent addiction and probably some intravenous use of drugs. Kidneys probably starting to degenerate from phenacetin in Empirin®.[12,13]
1971-1973	66-68	Severe, intermittent abuse of codeine, Valium®, and Empirin®. Probably some injection abuse. Occasional falls due to Valium® abuse. Able to intermittently function with work at reasonably high level and even fly an airplane. Kidneys continue to deteriorate. Constipated due to narcotics. Poor dental care.
1973	68	Fell and sustained fractured hip requiring a metal pi for repair. Fall probably result of drug abuse.
1974-1976	68-70	Continuous intravenous abuse of codeine and probably Empirin®. Drugs supplied by physicians. Unable to walk due to hip problem and develops leg contractures. Work, hygiene, diet, and dental care deteriorate. Progressive renal failure and uremic poisoning.
April 7, 1976	70	Dies from kidney failure due to chronic phenacetin (found in Empirin®) abuse. Autopsy shows brain and heart in good condition for age, so HRH could have lived much longer and in better health had he not misused drugs.

III. Legal Aspects of Case

A. Facts Bearing on Case

1. Codeine and Empirin-Codeine® are narcotics whose control and distribution are regulated by the "Federal comprehensive drug Abuse Prevention Control Act of 1970. (Title 21, United States Code). Plain codeine is listed under this act as a Schedule II drug, and Empirin-Codeine® a Schedule III drug. Schedule II drugs have a high potential for abuse and may lead to dependence, but have an accepted medical use with restrictions in the United states.

2. The Law clearly states that if a Schedule II drug is dispensed to a person by a practitioner other than a pharmacist and in other than an emergency situation, it shall be prescribed on a triplicate prescription. The use of the drug must be for an accepted medical use which in the case of codeine is only for pain.

IV. References

1. Tennant FS Jr. Development of Addiction to Prescribed Narcotics. Calif Soc for Treatment of Alcoholism and other Drug Dependencies 3:3, 1978.

2. Himmelsbach CK. Studies of Certain Addiction Characteristics of (a) Dihydromorphine ("Paramorphan"), (b) Dihydrodesoxymorphine-D ("Desomorphine"), (c) Dihydrodesoxycodeine-C ("Desocodeine"), and (d) Methyldihydromorphinone ("Metopon"). J Pharmacol Exp Ther 67:239-249, 1939.

3. Seevers MH and Feiffer CC. A Study of the Analgesia, Subjective Depression, and Euphoria Produced by Morphine, Heroin, Dilaudid, and Codeine in the Normal Human Subject. J Pharmacol Exp Ther 56:166-187, 1936.

4. Lasagna L and Beecher HK. The Analgesic Effectiveness of Codeine and Meperidine Demerol). J Pharmacol Exp Ther 112:306, 1954.

5. Himmelsbach CK and Andrews HL. Studies on Codeine Addiction. II. Studies of Physical Dependence of Codeine. Public Health Rep Suppl 158:11-17, 1940.

6. Kay DC, Gorodetzky CW, and Martin WR. Comparative Effects of Codeine and Morphine in Man. J Pharmacol Exp Ther 156:101-106, 1967.

7. Jaffee JH and Martin WR. Narcotic Analgesics and Antagonists: The Pharmacologic Basis of Therapeutics (Goodman CS and Gilman a eds) The MacMillan Co., New York, New York, 1975, pp 245-284.

8. Tennant FS Jr. Outpatient Treatment and Outcome of Prescription Drug Abuse. Arch Intern Med (In Press).

9. Shuster MM, Lewin MC. Needle Tracks in Narcotic Addicts. New York St J Med 68:3129-3134, 1968.

10. Young AW, Rosenberg FR. Cutaneous Stigmas of Heroin Addiction. Arch Derm 104:80-86, 1971.

11. Tennant FS Jr. Complications of Propoxyphene abuse. Arch Intern Med 132:191-194, 1973.

12. Murray T and Goldberg M. Chronic Interstitial Nephritis: Etiologic Factors. Ann Intern Med 82:453-459, 1975.

13. Nordenfelt D. Deaths from Renal Failure in Abusers of Phenacetin Containing Drugs. Acta Med Scand 191:11-16, 1972.

THE METHODIST HOSPITAL TEXAS MEDICAL CENTER

6516 BERTNER * HOUSTON, TEXAS 77025 * (713) 790-3311 * CABLE: METHHOSP

DEPARTMENT OF

PATHOLOGY (REPORT) APRIL 6, 1976

Dr. Jack L. Titus dictating notes for the record on the case of Mr. Howard R. Hughes.

Shortly after 9:00 AM on Monday, April 5, 1976, Dr. Henry McIntosh, and Mr. Ted Bowen informed mem confidentially that Mr. Howard R. Hughes was to arrive at The Methodist Hospital shortly after noon on that date in a critically ill state. Reportedly he was being transferred to The Methodist Hospital from Acapulco, Mexico. I was asked to arrange the most marked confidentiality of any and all laboratory work related to his case and, at the same time, expedite any and all laboratory work because of his critical illness. Appropriate arrangements were made for that aspect of his hospitalization. The patient was to be admitted under the pseudonym of John T. Conover.

Subsequently at approximately 2:00 PM on Monday, April 5, 1976 I received a call from Mr. Ted Bowen who had just been informed that the hospital conveyance and the physician who had gone to meet the plane bringing Mr. Hughes to Houston had found that he had died in route. The body was being transported to The Methodist Hospital morgue until appropriate arrangements, particularly from a legal standpoint, as well as from the family standpoint, could be made.

At 2:50 PM on Monday, April 5, 1976 Mr. Ted Bowen and I were at the morgue dock of The Methodist Hospital when a Methodist Hospital ambulance arrived. Dr. Robert Berglund, Chief Medical Resident, a hospital nurse, Mr. Jay Dixon, and Mr. Len Stom accompanied the body of an elderly white male. These individuals stated that this was the body of the man known as Mr. John T. Conover, who was stated to be Mr. Howard Hughes.

Under our supervision (that is, Mr. Ted Bowen and myself) the body was moved to the morgue of The Methodist Hospital. At 3:00 PM on Monday, April 5, 1976, in The Methodist Hospital morgue, I performed a brief external examination of the body reported to be that of Mr. Howard Hughes. The findings were those of an elderly white male with gray hair, somewhat thinned, and a gray beard. The body appeared remarkably emaciated and dehydrated. The estimated length of the body would be about 6'2." A plastic intrave catheter was present in the left antecubital fossa and the left arm was taped to a towel covered board. The body had been covered with a yellow blanket. The eyes were open and the pupils dilated and fixed. Although there were contractures of moderate degree of the knees, it should be noted that there was no evidence of rigor mortis in in any of the skeletal muscles of the body. Likewise, there was no evidence of livor mortis. Based upon the information that the body came from the cabin of airplane at appropriate environmental temperatures, was transported immediately by an ambulance at appropriate environmental temperatures, and this examination done essentially immediately upon arrival of the body at The Methodist Hospital morgue, it is my firm opinion that death occurred less than three hours prior to the time of my examination. Other physicians present at the time of this brief initial examination included Doctors Malcolm H. McGavran, Robert Berglund, Roberto J. Bayardo, and Henry D. McIntosh. Other observers were Mr. Ted Bowen, Mr. Larry Mathis and Mr. Ray Henderson, the latter most being an autopsy technician of the Pathology Service of The Methodist Hospital. The opinion as to the preliminary estimate as to death having occurred less than three hours prior to the examination at 3:00 PM on April 5, 1976 was concurred in by Doctors McGavran and Bayard, the other two pathologists present.

Pending notification of next of kin, the arrival at the hospital of the attending physician who accompanied Mr. Hughes to Houston, and assessment of the legal aspects of the situation, the body was placed in a body cooler in the morgue of The Methodist Hospital. Security measures were arranged for to be maintained continuously throughout the remainder of the day with Mr. Ray Henderson, Autopsy Technician, in constant attendant a designated administrator of The Methodist Hospital in constant attendance, and a security officer of The Methodist Hospital in constant attendance.

At approximately 3:15 to 3:30 PM on April 5, 1976 I met in Mr. Bowen's office along with other physicians and administrators of The Methodist Hospital with the individuals that had accompanied Mr. Hughes to Houston. These included Dr. Lawrence Chaffin, Dr. Wilbur Thain and Mr. John Holmes. In our preliminary interview, from a medical standpoint the salient features, in my opinion, of Mr. Hughes' medical history included the following:

1. An extraordinary reluctance to permit the usual medical evaluations.
2. A history of a fracture of the left hip in August, 1973 which was repaired surgically in London, England.
3. Some propensity to self-medicate with a variety of proprietary medications, including aspirin and phenacetin containing compounds.
4. Regarding the apparent final illness, Drs. Chaffin and Thain reported that from their limited knowledge, Mr. Hughes had been reported to them as not having been eating nor drinking well for approximately the last three weeks.

In addition, he apparently had increasing malaise. Over the past two or three days of life, particularly the past 24-36 hours, he developed some confusion. Somewhat suddenly and unexpectedly on Sunday evening, April 4, he developed a shock-like state for which he was treated with intravenous fluids. In recognition of the apparent sudden worsening of his condition, the decision was made to transfer him to Houston for further care as soon as arrangements could be made. Dr. Chaffin, Dr. Thain and Mr. Holmes told us that in his seriously ill state, apparently nearly comatose, he was put in a private jet with the aforementioned three gentlemen in attendance and transferred to Houston.

During most of the flight from Acapulco, Mexico to Houston his condition remained essentially unchanged; that is, unresponsive with intravenous fluids running and oxygen being administered. Sometime after the plane had passed Brownsville, Texas there was progressive loss of all vital signs so that at the time of beginning let down in Houston, all vital signs had ceased. Dr. Thain noted the time to be 1:27 PM, CST. Subsequent events are as described in the foregoing paragraphs with the transportation of the body to The Methodist Hospital and our observations upon arrival there.

Having determined from the foregoing that (1) this patient, reported to be Mr. Howard Hughes, had died in Texas; (2) that the plane bearing is body had landed in the jurisdiction of the Harris County Medical Examiner; (3) that death had occurred at approximately 1:30 PM, CST on April 5, 1976; and (4) that no physician licensed in Texas was in attendance prior to death, it was clear that the Medical Examiner for Harris County must be contacted. Therefore at 4:00 PM I was able to reach Dr. Ethel Erickson, Deputy Medical Examiner of Harris County as Dr. Joseph Jachimczyk, Medical Examiner for Harris County was at that moment out of the city. I explained the entirety of the situation to Dr. Erickson. I indicated to Dr. Erickson that the attending physicians were present and in addition contact had been made with the next of kin, Mrs. F. Lummis of Houston, who is an aunt of Mr. Hughes. Her sone, Mr. Will Lummis, an attorney in Houston, representing his mother with power of attorney for his mother, came to the hospital to handle the immediate funeral arrangements.

After discussion among all the parties concerned and further discussions with Dr. Erickson, at about 800 PM on April 5, 1976 Dr. Jachimczyk, who had returned to town, and Dr. Erickson met with Mr. Lummis, Dr. Thain, Mr. Holmes, Mr. Larry Mathis, and me. Dr. Jachimczyk indicated the necessity for an autopsy. As a courtesy to the family of Mr. Hughes and to the Hughes interests, he indicated that if an appropriate autopsy permit were given by the next of kin, and, if the Pathology Department of The Methodist Hospital were willing to perform a complete autopsy and thereafter, complete a proper death certificate, the Medical Examiner's office would consider that the legal requirements of the situation were satisfied. Parenthetically, it may be noted that this is the usual and customary practice for Houston patients who are DOA at Houston hospitals. After these consultations, Mr. Will Lummis indicated he would discuss the question of an autopsy further with his mother, but was certain that he could return the next morning, that is, Tuesday, April 6, 1976, to sign an autopsy permit which would authorize pathologists at The Methodist Hospital to conduct a complete autopsy on the body reported to be Mr. Howard Hughes.

On Tuesday morning, April 6, 1976, Mr. Lummis signed the usual Methodist Hospital autopsy permit from which was duly witnessed. Hospital legal counsel agreed it was appropriate permission. Dr. Jachimczyk was informed that a proper autopsy permit had been obtained and that a complete autopsy would begin at about 1:00 PM on Tuesday, April 6, 1976. The autopsy would be carried out by myself in concert with Doctors Malcolm McGavran and Roberto Bayardo. Dr. Jachimczyk and Dr. Erickson were invited to be present as knowledgeable colleagues whose expertise was deemed appropriate. In addition, as is usually the case, the attending physicians, Drs., Thain, Chaffin, and McIntosh, were asked to attend. Arrangements were made to obtain specific identification by usual methodologies including finger printing, total body x-rays, and preparation of a dental chart. Following these arrangements in view of a valid autopsy permission signed by the appropriate next of kin arrangements for clear identification of the individual to be autopsied, and appropriate consultation with the Harris County Medical Examiner's office, the autopsy described in the protocol that follows was done. The autopsy number assigned to this case is N-76-92.

This concludes the notes preliminary to the formal autopsy protocol and report on case N-76-92, Mr. Howard Hughes. The time is 5:00 PM, April 6, 1976, when this record is dictated from notes made over the past 24 hours or so.

Jack L. Titus, M.D., Ph.D.

Chief, Pathology Service

The Methodist Hospital

FORENSIC PATHOLOGY

ATTORNEY AT LAW

CHIEF MEDICAL EXAMINER

OFFICE OF THE MEDICAL EXAMINER

OF HARRIS COUNTY

HARRIS COUNTY COOURT HOUSE

HOUSTON, TEXAS 77002

April 10, 1976

TOXICOLOGICAL EXAMINATION

RE: Howard R. Hughes

CASE NUMBER: N-76-92

LABORATORY RESULTS

Alcohol = Negative (Cerebrospinal fluid)

Barbiturates = Negative (Blood)

Acetylsalicylic acid = Negative (Blood)

Drug Screen = Negative (Blood, Urine, Liver and Stomach Contents)

Phenacetin = Negative (Blood, Urine, Liver and Stomach Contents)

Narcotics = 0.196 mg. % Codeine (Blood)

4.8 mg. % Codeine (Bile)

6.6 mg. % Codeine (Urine)

0.7mg % Codeine (Liver)

2.2 mg. % Codeine (Stomach Contents)

Blood Group = "A"

The Strange Medical Saga of Howard Hughes

Joseph A Jachimczyk, M.D., J.D.

Chief Medical Examiner

Larry D. Hobbs

Assistant Toxicologist

September 10, 1978

THE METHODIST HOSPITAL TEXAS MEDICAL CENTER

6516 BERTNER * HOUSTON, TEXAS 77025 * (713) 790-3311 * CABLE: METHHOSP

DEPARTMENT OF

PATHOLOGY (REPORT) APRIL 7, 1976

Henry D. McIntosh, M.D.

6516 Bertner

Houston, Texas 77030

Dear Doctor McIntosh,

The following are the preliminary anatomic diagnoses on Howard R. Hughes, autopsy number N-76-92. Mr. Hughes reportedly died at 1:27 PM CST on April 5, 1976 and was dead on arrival at The Methodist Hospital at 2:50 PM CST, April 5, 1976. The autopsy was performed on April 6, 1976, beginning at 1:30 PM.

Cause of Death:

Chronic renal failure due to chronic interstitial nephritis with papillary necrosis.

Major Diagnoses:

1. Granular atrophy of kidneys (total weight 200 grams) with necrosis most of renal papillae.
2. Adenofibromatous hyperplasia prostate with prominent median bar partially obstruction urethra.
3. Moderate stricture urethral meatus.
4. Renal failure.
5. Emaciation and dehydration.
6. Generalized osteoporosis.

Additional Findings:

1. Fibrotic apical scars both lungs and old, fibrotic left pleural adhesions (history of prior left thoracic injury).
2. Metallic pin left hip from repair of prior fracture.
3. Separation left acromio-clavicular joint with edema and hematoma left shoulder.
4. Chronic peptic gastric ulcer at incisura angularis.
5. Single focus of grade 3 atherosclerotic narrowing (60% luminal narrowing) in mid left anterior descending coronary artery; focal calcification medial aspect mitral valve annulus.
6. Focal complex atherosclerotic lesions aorta (grade 2 atherosclerotic disease).
7. Adenoma (2 cm.) right lobe of thyroid.
8. Single left vertebral artery.
9. Moderate dilatation occipital portions of lateral cerebral ventricles.
10. Cylindroma left parietal scalp.
11. Multiple needle punctures and ecchymoses forearms

Henry D. McIntosh, M.D.

April 7, 1976
Page Two

Toxicologic and histologic studies are in progress. As soon as these studies are completed, the final autopsy report will be available.

Sincerely yours,

Jack L. Titus, M.D., Ph.D.
Chief, Pathology Service
The Methodist Hospital

JLT/bjs
Cc: Wilbur S. Thain, M.D.
Lawrence Chaffin, M.D.

THE METHODIST HOSPITAL TEXAS MEDICAL CENTER

6516 BERTNER * HOUSTON, TEXAS 77025 * (713) 790-3311 * CABLE: METHHOSP

AUTOPSY PROTOCOL

N-76-92

Howard R. Hughes

70 years old

Male Caucasian

EXTERNAL EXAMINATION

The body is that of an aged, cachectic, Caucasian male weighing 42 kilograms and measuring 185 cm. The skin "tents" when elevated. The hair and beard are grey. The sclera are clear, the corneas have arcus senilis bilaterally, the irides are brown, the pupils are RR and e at 4 mm. The auditory canals are clear. A 212 cm oval, centrally ulcerated, nodule is present on the left parietal scalp. The hair surrounding this has been trimmed. The oral cavity and pharynx are clear. The teeth are carious (see attached dental report). The trachea is midline. The thyroid is not palpable.

The left supra and infraclavicular fossae as well as the left shoulder and upper arm and posterior axillary fold are modestly swollen, edematous, and discolored a bluish-grey. A left acromio-clavicular separation is palpable with overriding of the clavicle. The remaining skin of the anterior chest is unremarkable. Multiple recent needle punctures and recent ecchymoses are present on both forearms. The abdomen is scaphoid. The penis is circumcised; urethral meatus is small measuring 4 mm. The testes are intrascrotal. The groins and perineum are without lesions. The anus is patent and without lesions.

A 17 cm linear scar is present on the left hip from the level of the pubic symphysis distally. The remainder of the thighs and legs show bilateral 15-20° flexion contractures of the knees. A metallic pin in the left hip is demonstrated by radiologic examination.

Examination of the back shows a distinct dorsal scoliosis with the curvature to the right, and depressed white scars overlying the left mid scapula and running laterally and inferiorly to the mid axillary line at the level of the costal margin. Six, 1.5-2.5 cm superficial, centrally crusted ulcers of the skin over the sacrum and adjacent iliosacral areas are present.

INTERNAL EXAMINATION

Subcutaneous adipose tissue is scant to absent and 2 mm in thickness over the mid abdomen.

The diaphragms are both at the level of the 6th interspace. The right pleural cavity contains 30 ml of serous fluid, the left 20 ml of like fluid and the pericardium 50 ml of clear serous fluid. The peritoneum is dry. All organs are normally situated. The left pleural cavity is partially obliterated by fibrous adhesions.

Heart

The heart weighs 340 grams. The right and left ventricular thickness are 10 mm and 3 mm, respectively. The tricuspid, pulmonic, mitral, and aortic rings measure 13.5, 8.7, 12.4 and 9.2 cm. The mitral ring is focally calcified medially. No valvular lesions save fenestrations are noted. No epicardial, myocardial or endocardial lesions are noted. The left coronary artery is dominant. Mild to focally moderate coronary atherosclerosis is present with a single focus of 60% luminal narrowing in the mid portion of the left anterior descending artery

Vessels

The aorta is minimally involved by nonulcerated atheromatous plaques in the ascending arch and descending portions. The abdominal aorta distal to the renal vessels shows 4 ulcerated plaques with attached fibrinous thrombi. The great vessels of the neck and abdominal branches arise in their usual anatomic positions. The renal arteries are patent and show minimal atherosclerosis. The pulmonary arteries are patent and without evidence of thromboemboli. The inferior vena cava, renal and hepatic veins are patent and without lesions. The portal and splenic veins are grossly normal.

Lungs

The right lung weighs 300 grams and the left lung 390 grams. Save for the previously described fibrous adhesions and bilateral fibrous apical scars, no lesions are found. The tracheobronchial tree and larynx are without lesions.

Liver

The liver weighs 1180 grams and is grossly of normal appearance. Multiple transections show no lesions. The bile ducts and gallbladder are without lesions.

Pancreas

The pancreas weighs 100 grams and is grossly normal.

Spleen

The spleen weighs 110 grams and is grossly normal.

Adrenals

The adrenals weigh 7 and 8 grams, left and right, and are grossly normal.

Thyroid

The thyroid weighs 25 grams. The lower pole of the left lobe contains a single, sharply delimited, 2 cm, tan nodule. The remainder of this lobe and the right are grossly normal.

Parathyroids

The parathyroids are not grossly enlarged.

Testis

The testis weigh 20 and 22 grams, right and left. They are grossly normal.

Kidney

The kidneys, right and left, weigh 90 and 110 grams. The capsules are adherent and when stripped, show irregularly granular cortical surfaces with interspersed linear depressions. Upon transection the cortices are markedly thinned, averaging 2 mm in thickness. The medullae are firm and partially replaced by grey fibrous tissue. All of the renal papillae are shrunken and the residual papillae lined by whitish streaks. The calyces, renal pelvis and ureters are not dilated.

Prostate

The prostate is enlarged, approximate 3x, and evidences nodular hyperplasia with a prominent median bar.

Urinary Bladder

The urinary bladder is filled with approximately 250 ml of cloudy yellow urine. The wall is trabeculated. No mucosal abnormalities are noted. The ureteral orifices are not dilated.

Esophagus

No abnormalities.

Stomach

A linear, 2 x 0.5 cm, chronic peptic ulcer is present on the lesser curvature of the stomach at the incisura.

Duodenum and Small Bowel

No abnormalities.

Large Intestine

Sigmoid diverticula are present. No mucosal or mural lesions are noted.

Bones

The vertebral bodies are moderately osteoporotic as are the ribs and sternum.

Brain and Spinal Cord

The dura is intact and no evidences of epidural or subdural hematomas, recent or remote, are found. The brain weighs 1540 grams. The cortical surfaces show no lesions. The basilar cerebral vessels are with usual anatomic distribution with the exception that only one vertebral artery is present, situated on the left. No aneurysms are noted at any of the bifurcations. Atheromatous involvement is minimal. No evidences of cingulate, uncial or cerebellar tonsillar herniation is present.

Multiple 0.5+1.5 cm tick transections of the cerebrum, cerebellum and brain stem show no abnormalities of the cortex, white matter, thalamus cerebellum, pons, or medulla. Modest dilatation o f the occipital poles of the lateral ventricle, aqueduct of Silvius and 4th ventricle are not dilated. The spinal cord shows no gross abnormalities.

Malcolm H. McGavran, M.D.

Chief, Anatomic Pathology

Jack L. Titus, M.D., Ph.D.

Chief, Pathology Service

The Methodist Hospital

MICROSCOPIC EXAMINATION

The salient abnormalities corroborating and extending the gross findings are:

Kidneys

The renal papillae are shrunken and fibrotic showing extensive loss of collecting tubules with residual peritubular hyalinization and both interstitial and intratubular deposits of urates and calcium. No active acute inflammatory process is present, and no frank recent necrosis is found. The arcuate and interlobular arteries show modest to marked fibrosis subintimal thickening. Extensive zones of obsolete, totally fibrotic glomeruli and scarring are present with mild to modest lymphoid interstitial inflammatory infiltrate. Acute pyelonephritis is not present.

Prostate

Nodular hyperplasia, predominantly adenomatous is present. A microfocus of well differentiated adenocarcinoma is also present.

Urinary Bladder

Mild chronic cystitis is present.

Pancreas

Mild centrilobular ductal dilation with retained secretion is present.

Bone Marrow

The marrow is minimally hypoplastic. The vertebral bodies evidence modest osteoporosis. Evidences of osteitis fibrosa re not found.

Skin

The lesion of the left parietal scalp is an eccrine adenoid cystic adenocarcinoma (Cylindroma).

Thyroid

The nodule in the left lower pole is a follicular adenoma.

Stomach

The ulcer is chronic with fibrous replacement of part of the muscularis.

Lungs

The apical scars are without evidence of active inflammatory or granulomatous component. The remainder of the samples show no evidence of pneumonia or passive congestion.

Sections of the heart, liver, adrenals, brain, pituitary, bone marrow, spleen show no abnormalities.

Malcolm H. McGavran, M.D.

Chief, Anatomic Pathology

Jack L. Titus, M.D., Ph.D.

Chief, Pathology Service

The Methodist Hospital

Microscopic of Brain - CNS

Cerebrum: Slight fibrosis of leptomeninges. Precentral cortical grey matter really well preserved motor nervous. There is no evidence of accelerated involutional changes of the cerebrum cortex.

Diencephalon and brain stem: Thalamus and inferior olivary nucleus show hypertrophic astrocytes (Alzheimer type II), consistent with metabolic changes.

Spinal cord: not remarkable.

Diagnosis: No diagnosis.

M. Suzuki

OPERATING MEMORANDUM

October 2, 1958

Subject: Instructions from HRH regarding securing and processing prescriptions

If there is a prescription required by either HRH or Mrs. Hughes, then the following procedures should be followed:

If any prescription has to be taken to the drugstore to be filled and there is a reasonable amount of time, then use a public messenger service. Have him deliver the prescription to the drugstore and have the druggist put the price of his services on the bill and pay the messenger on the spot. When we arrive to pick up the prescription, then we will pay cash for the total amount of the bill, including the amount of the messenger service. There are to be no prescriptions charged under any circumstances, we should pay cash at all times. All prescription should be telephoned in, if possible. If they insist on mailing a copy later, then OK, as that is better than having it taken to the drugstore originally. If it is a triplicate type prescription (for narcotics) then use a public messenger service, without any contact with any of our personal and without them knowing who it is for or who the name of the company is.

If the prescription is for HRH, then Roy should fill and supervise the prescription and then have Harris deliver it. If Harris isn't available, then Roy should do both jobs. If that isn't convenient, then Kay should do it. If that is impossible, then use a staff man. Bill Gay would never be involved in any way that would break the isolation of him. Do not use any of his people, that is, any people connected with Bill in any way, under any circumstances. As a last resort – timewise – use a driver that is as close to the drugstore where the prescription is located as possible.

When the call comes into the office following the doctors call to Mrs. Hughes and it is something that can be telephoned in, then OK. Try to prevail on the doctor not to require a confirmation of the prescription. It would be well to put the prescription in Mrs. Melba Doss' name, as Mrs. Hughes would like that better than using another name she doesn't know.

If Kay or Bill is masterminding the deal, then have Roy handle the delivering and filling of the prescription (Make sure that nobody knows the name or address that is connected with the prescription, or the company's name). When you are talking to the messenger service, tell him: "This is Dr. Hawkin's secretary calling, (do not use Roy's or any of our people's name) would you please go to such and such address and pick up a prescription and take it to Horton & Converse drugstore at such and such address. They will pay you and just put the amount on our bill." Then, Roy should go over and supervise the filling of the prescription. If Roy is out of town, then maybe before he goes he should leave instructions with Kay or Bill, or both, as to the name of the drugstore and the clerk who does this service for him and also get the name of the messenger service from Roy, as Roy has been doing this for some time now. Roy (or Kay) should remain at the drugstore and monitor the operation there like Roy has been doing – or like Roy instructs Kay to. If Bill is handling this should then have a man operating under his (Bill's) instruction at the drugstore. This should, of course, not be anyone connected with Bill.

Now, if there is such a time emergency that we do not have time to go to this particular drugstore that Roy has been using and also, in case there is such a time element that we do not want to wait, we should check a drugstore ahead of time that is in the vicinity of the hotel (not Schwab's or the Beverly Wilshire Hotel's or any drugstore that is used by the movie people). If we deviate from the store that Roy has been using, then do not use Roy at all. We really should have two drugstores located, one for day-time use and another for night-time use. Roy should not be used in a way that would bring him in physical contact with anything contaminating. Do not ever use Roy in a dry-run operation, in other words, if you are trying out a fake operation, have two teams, which would be used when we use the alternate drugstores that we are going to select. The number one team should consist of Kay alone. He will do the telephoning and also the pick up. The number two team should consist of Bill Gay to do the telephoning and another man, to be selected by Bill, to do the pick up.

In selecting a name to go on the prescription, if it is for me, then use the names that Roy has been using. I think that has been Mrs. Lee Murrin. If it is for Mrs. Hughes, then I would use the name of her aunt, Mrs. Malba Doss, if it is a prescription that can be telephoned in. If it is one of those triplicate type prescriptions, then I would use Mrs. Lee Murrin. She knows that I use Mrs. Lee Murrin all the time and she would not be offended over that.

Roy should try to arrange, through the man that he knows at his drugstore, to get names of two or three other men that stand other shifts that might be trusted to follow our procedures so when we need something at a time when Roy's regular man is off duty, we can work through these other men on shift. If the prescription involves Jean and not HRH, then do not use Roy in the delivery operation at all, just use him for telephoning and do not have him go to the drugstore to supervise the operation at all. Also, do not use Harris fro the delivery. If time permits the use of Roy's drugstore, then use Roy in the supervision and either the number one group (Kay alone) of the number two group (Bill and one other man) in the execution and delivery. If time does not permit te use of the drugstore that Roy uses, then we use the two different groups and DO NOT use Roy in any phase of the operation at all. In other words, if we have to use the two alternate drugstores for any reason, Roy or Harris will not be used at all.

As this thing goes now, we have three people that can do the telephoning – Roy, Bill and Kay, and we have two people who can do the pick up and delivery – Kay and Bill's man. If it is for HRH then Roy will do the whole thing, telephoning, supervision, and delivery. This is, of course, assuming that time will permit this and if time does not permit it, then Roy will telephone and supervise and either Harris, Kay or Bill's man will make the pick up, in that order. If the time element is a further consideration, then the additional man (the ones that Roy will set up) will do the supervision. If time is a further element, then we move into the alternate drugstore that has been selecte4d and from there, Roy and Harris will not be used at all, the telephonic conversation will be done by either Kay or Bill.

If the prescription is for Jean, then Roy isn't used at all. We follow the same identical procedures as above, same procedures as used for HRH, except the name will be changed and Roy will not have any physical contact or participation, as the two groups will handle. This, of course, also excludes Johnny, Harris, George of the third man.

There is one exception that Roy might be used in the procedure for getting a prescription set up for Jean and that is, if by any remote chance, and I certainly can't think of any reason that this would happen, both Kay and Bill are unavailable at the same time, then I want Roy to participate ONLY in the telephonic supervision from his regular telephones, which would be either his own telephone at home or the one at his office. I don't want Roy ever using any other telephone in his procedures and telephoning except the two mentioned.

"I want absolutely nothing that I have said here tonight in connection with any of these instructions to alter, diminish, subtract from or affect in any way the Bill Gay isolation program in any slightest detail whatsoever."

Daily Log		
Sunday Oct. 31 ,71	10:45 am	Chair, screening "THE KILLERS," THE GOOD GUYS AND THE BAD GUYS" completed reels 1&2.
	1:10 pm	Bed/ Washed and bandage wound
	1:30	B/R
	1:45	Chair, screening "THE HELL WITH HEROES". Inst: don't ship and of the movies he has cleared yet, until he has a chance to look at them this evening.
	2:20	Food: Chicken and one dessert only.
	3:30	Finished eating. Finish screening "THE HELL WITH HEROES" AND "SPARTACUS". OK to return these two films.
	5:50	B/R
	6:05	Chair, resumed screening "THE GOOD GUYS AND BAD GUYS."
	6:55	B/R
	7:10	Chair
	8:20	Chicken and dessert
	11:00	Finished eating
	11:30	B/R
	11:55	Chair
Monday Nov. 1, 71		Completed "GOOD GUYS & BAD GUYS" & "WALK ON THE WILD SIDE". OK to return. Also screened "HOTEL".
	5:00 AM	Finished CASTLE KEEP. OK to return. note: All of the NY films can be returned.

	5:15	B/R
	5:45	Bed
	5:55	B/R
	9:55	Bed, Asleep
	3:45 PM	Awake, B/R
	4:40	Chair
	5:30	Screening "THE KILLERS."
	6:00	Food: chicken
	7:30	Finished eating and asleep in chair
Tues. 11/2/71	12:05 AM	B/AR
	12:40	Bed & change dressing
	1:05	B/R
	1:50	Chair
	4:00	B/R
	4:30	Chair
	5:00	Started screening THE KILLERS.
	5:40	Started eating
	8:00	Finished eating. Finished THE KILLERS.
	8:05	B/R Shower
	8:55	Bed. Changed dressing
	9:20	B/R
	9:40	Chair
	10:55	Screening REAP THE WILD WIND.
	12:45 PM	B/R
	1:15	Chair, resumed screening "REAP THE WILD WIIND", competed reels 1,2,3 & part of reel 4. Screening "THE KILLERS".
	3:10	B/R. 4½ BB's
	3:30	Chair, resumed screening "THE KILLERS". Completed.
	4:30	Food: Chicken & dessert. Screened

		"THE KILLERS" again.
	6:15	Finished eating. Finished "REAP THE WILD WIND".
Tues. Dec. 8, 71	1: 00 AM	B/R
	1:10	Bed
	3:10	B/R & Shower.
	4:10	Chair
	6:45	Chicken & 10 Indians.
	7:55	Finished chicken
	8:10	8c 34 left?
	9:00	B/R
	9:30	Chair
	11:30	Norman & Homer in
	12:30 PM	out
	12:25	B/R
	1:05	Chair. Screened "TENSION AT TABLE ROCK"
	1:30	Food
	3:30	Finished complete meal & 10 Indians.
	4:05	2½ BB's. B/R.
	5:00	Bed. Asleep
	9:45	B/R
	11:00	Bed
Wednesday Dec. 8, 71	1:55 AM	B/R
	2:55	Chair
	8:55	Food
	4:00	B/R
	4:35	Chair
	5:10	Food
	6:25	Finished chicken and 10 Indians.
	6:55	B/R INSTRUCTIONS: DO NOT PUT THE SPONGE RUBBER INSIDE OF ANY PILLOW CASE—IN FACT HE DOES NOT WANT ANYTHING

		WHATSOEVER PUT INSIDE THE PILLOW CASE. HE WANTS THE PILLOW CASE TO BE TREATED AS IF IT WERE A SINGLE LAYER OF MATERIAL.
	7:30	Chair
	8:50	B/R
	9:20	Chair Screening "DEADLIER THAN THE MALE"
	11:00	B/R
	11:50	Chair, Started eating. 4bb.
	1:45 PM	XX Finished eating. S-1-1-1. B/r.
	2:10	Chair. 2bb. Screening TEN LITTLE INDIANS.
	4:30	B/R
	5:15	Bed. Asleep?
Thursday Dec. 9, 71	1:50 AM	Awake, B/R, shower
	3:35	Chair & R 1 "10 Indians"
	4:40	B/R
	5:10	Chair
	5:55	Chicken & R 1 "10 Indians"
	7:10	Finished chicken only & Reels 2 & 3 or "10 Indians"
	8:10	B/R
	8:45	Chair. Screened reels 1,2 "DEADLIER THAN THE MALE"
	10:20	B/R
	11:00	Chair. Finished DEADLIER THAN THE MALE.
	Noon	B/R
	12:30 PM	Chair. Screening TEN LITTLE INDIANS.

		Started eating.
	2:30	Finished eating. Screening THE WRECKING CREW.
	3:15	B/R
	3:30	Chair
Saturday July 8, 72	4:00 AM	B/R "I'M VERY SICK".
	5:30	Chair
	7:10	B/R
	7:50	Chair
	9:00	B/R
	10:15	Chair
	11:00	Screening "I WANTED WINGS" reels 3&4.
	12:15 PM	Started eating chicken & dessert
	2:10	Finished eating complete meal
	2:15	Screening "I WANTED WINGS" again
	3:50	Norman in to bandage the left heel.
	4:30	B/R & Big E. (2)
	7:45	Chair
	9:00	B/R
	9:15	Chair
	11:05	B/R
7/9/72	3:00 AM	B/R
	3:45	Chair – "APPOINTMENT WITH A SHADOW". Completed.
	5:35	B/R
	5:50	Chair – "DEAN RUN". Completed.
	7:15	Dessert only
	8:50	Finished dessert
	9:15	6 BB's. "A MAN COULD GET KILLED". INSTRUCTIONS: Please refrain from placing box containing

		Kleenex on the square table to the loft that contains the "CREW MANUALS".
	9:50	B/R
	10:30	Bed & Asleep.
	6:15 PM	B/R & awake
	7:00	Norman changed dressing
	8:00	"Rickard can pull a shift alone in one week"
	9:10	Chair
Monday July 10, 1972	12:40 AM	B/AR
	1:30	Chair. INSTRUCTIONS: When he has designated a time to eat, always notify him 10 minutes prior to that time, especially if he is dozing, so he can start setting his table. He wants us to find larger napkins for him to use in setting his table, similar or even larger than the ones he used in Managua.
	6:00 AM	Eating chicken. Finished chicken & "A MAN COULD GET KILLED".
	12:10 PM	Dessert & "AIRPORT"
	2:35	Norman changed dressing
	4:15	B/R
	4:45	Bed and asleep
7/11/72	3:10 AM	B/R
	4:00	Bed
	7:15	B/R
	9:00	Chair
	10:00	B/R
	12:05 PM	Chicken – screening

		"AIRPORT"
	3:15	Finished dessert finished screening "AIRPORT"Continued
Monday Sept. 25, 1972	To Chester:	Should filing be postponed until Oct. 10. What is the maximum time beyond Oct. 10. What did the Federal Agency say about his (HPH) explanation of the 10 million.
	To Holliday:	How does HPH) benefit personally or how does the Co. benefit whether the stock is sold this year or not. Explain your message of 9/20 in a different manner.
	To Real:	Congratulations on 5135 deal. Wants it pickled. Do not move it or any other planes to Van Nuys hangar. To whom do you think we can sublease Van Nuys hangar or parts of it to? Do not sell the D-H. Grab Richfield Oil offer but try to persuade them to shorten 3-month period & also to let us rent their entire hangar at Burbank.
	7:40 PM	Dessert – "THE ADVENTURERS" reel #1.
	10:45	Finished dessert
	11:30	B/R
Tues. Sept 26	1:15 AM	Dessert – "THE ADVENTURERS" reel #1.
	10:10 AM	B/R
	10:40	Bed & asleep

	10:45	B/R
	11:15	Chair. Screening THE ADVENTURERS. Completed. OK to return.
	3:00 PM	B/R
	3:50	Chair
	5:15	B/R
	7:25	Chair – "CLAY PIGEON" reel #1
	9:40	B/R
	11:55	Dessert "reels #2 & 3.
Wed. Sept 27	11:00 AM	Screening SUBTERRANEAN Completed. OK to return.
	1:00 PM	B/R
	1:25	Chair
	3:00	B/R
	3:15	Chair Screening ESCAPE FROM EAST BERLIN
	To Chester:	Would not going to #1 at this time generate publicity that we are seeking to avoid. He is against going at this time. Maybe next year. The press would demand an interview, etc.
	To Kay:	Will decide tonight or tomorrow on #1 hangar lease. Definitely wants options for 2-3 years. Wants high & low average temperatures by the month only for both #1 & Vancouver for next 6 months. Type on one sheet of paper showing comparisons.
	7:00 PM	Dessert – "ITALIAN JOB" reels 1 & 2.
	11:20	Finished dessert

Thurs, Sept 28	12:15 AM	B/R. Kay instructed to lease hangar at #1 with a series of 6-month options running up to 10 years. He does not want to share hangar because of the sophisticate air conditioning & dehumidifying equipment he plans to install.
Thurs. Feb. 1, 1973	2:45 AM	B/R
	3:00	Chair – "BLOWUP" reels 2 & 3. Completed.
	4:30	B/R
	4:45	Chair, screening "ROBERY UNDER ARMS". Completed.
	5:50	Started eating flakes. Screening "THE McMASTERS".
	9:00	Finished eating flakes & "THE McMASTERS"
	9:10	B/R
	9:35	Chair, screening "TAKE THE HIGH GROUND". OK to return. Reel one only.
	10:30	B/R
	10:45	Chair, screening "DEADLY ROULETTE".
	11:55	B/R
	12:25 PM	Chair
	1:35	B/R
	1:45	Chair
	4:00	Dessert only, screening DEADLY ROULETTE AGAIN
	6:00	Finished
	6:45	B/R "E"
Fri,	12:15 AM	Chair 6BB's

2/2/73		
	1:15	B/R
	1:45	Bed. Be sure to remind him to sign the bank notes when he awakens: but do not awaken him under any circumstances. They should reach bank by Monday morning Turn heat up on blanket as morning approaches.
	6:00 AM	B/R
	7:20	Bed & asleep. (3 BB's)
	4:40 PM	B/R
	5:25	Chair "THEY CAME TO ROB LAS VEGAS" 1½ reels.
	7:05	B/R
	7:45	Chair "THEY CAME TO ROB LAS VEGAS" 1½ reels.
	9:00	Chicken "reels 1 & 2.
	10:20	B/R
	10:45	Chair "reel 3.
	10:15	Flakes "STRANGERS ON A TRAIN" reels 1 & 2.
Sat Feb. 3	1:20 AM	Finished flakes " reel 3. Completed.
	2:00	B/R
	2:45	Chair, screening "POINT BLANK". Completed.
	4:40	Started eating cake.
	5:20	Screening "THE WRONG MAN". Part of reel 1 only. Screening "DOUBLE MAN". Completed.
	7:30 AM	Finished eating cake (3 pieces)
	8:00	B/D & Bidet
	8:45	Chair, given memos. Screening "CATCH A

		SPY"
	12:00 AM	B/R & Bidet
	1:15	Chair
	4:30	B/R 6 BB's 2 BB's later
	5:15	Bed & asleep
	10:30	B/R
	11:45	Bed
Sun. 2/4/73	4:10 AM	Awake and B/R
	4:35	Chair, said that he was not feeling every good. (6BB's)
	6:50	B/R
	7:05	Chair
	9:50	B/R
	10:20	Bed & asleep
	9:20 PM	B/R
	10:00	Chair "the third man" completed.
	????	Left for airport
	6:35	Returned to hotel
	7:00	Screening "TWO LANE BLACKTOP"
	7:55	Beef & Veg.
	10:05	Screening "THE BEGUILED"
	12:00 PM	Finished eating dessert & "THE BEGUILED"
	12:10	B/R (BM & shower)
	1:30	Bed & asleep. (7B's)
	4:45	Awake, B/R & to chair, screening "DEAD HEAT ON A MERRY-GO-ROUND" completed.
	7:15	Dessert
	8:50	Finished
	9:00	B/R
	9:25	Bed & asleep (3)
Fir. 6/29/73	12:50 AM	Awake & B/R
	1:10	Chair
	2:35	Screening "THE

		BEDFORD INCIDENT"
	3:05	Meat & vegetables
	5:35	Screening "FAIL SAFE"
	6:00	Dessert
	8:50	Bed & asleep
	12:35 PM	Awake & B/R
	1:00	Chair, asleep
	4:30	Awake & B/R
	5:10	Chair, screening "THE ESCAPE OF BIRDMEN" Complete.
	7:45	Beef & veg. & dessert
	9:00	Screening THE HIRED HAND
	10:30	B/R
	10:45	Chair. Screening YOU CAN'T WIN 'EM ALL completed.
Sat. 6/30/73	1:30 AM	B/R
	1:40	Chair
	2:00	Dessert only. Screening DEAD HEAT ON A MERRY-GO-ROUND
	4:20	B/R & back to chair
	5:30	Screening "COMPANY OF KILLERS"
	10:30	Started eating dessert. Completed "COMPANY OF KILLERS"
	10:45	Screening "DEVIL'S EIGHT"
	1:30 PM	Finished eating dessert & "DEVIL'S EIGHT"
	1:45	B/R
	2:20	Bed & asleep (7)
	5:30	B/R & back to bed
	8:10	B/R
	8:25	Bed
	9:35	Chair
	11:45	B/R

Sun. 7/1/73	12:10 AM	Chair, screening NEVER GIVE AN INCH, completed
	12:45	Beef & veg. & dessert
	3:30	Finished eating
	4:30	B/R
	6:20	Chair
	7:00	B/R
	7:30	Bed & asleep

INDEX

Other Books by Forest Tennant:

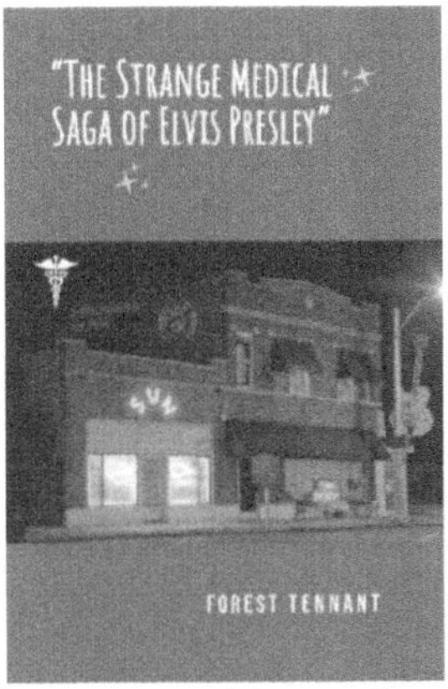

"THE STRANGE MEDICAL SAGA
OF ELVIS PRESLEY"
ISBN: 9781955934008
Library of Congress Control Number:
2021911718

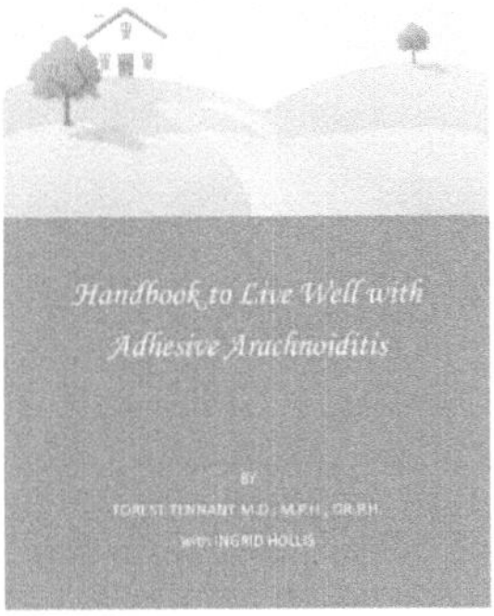

"HANDBOOK TO LIVE WELL WITH ADHESIVE
ARACHNOIDITIS"
ISBN: 978195934060
LOC: 2021912718

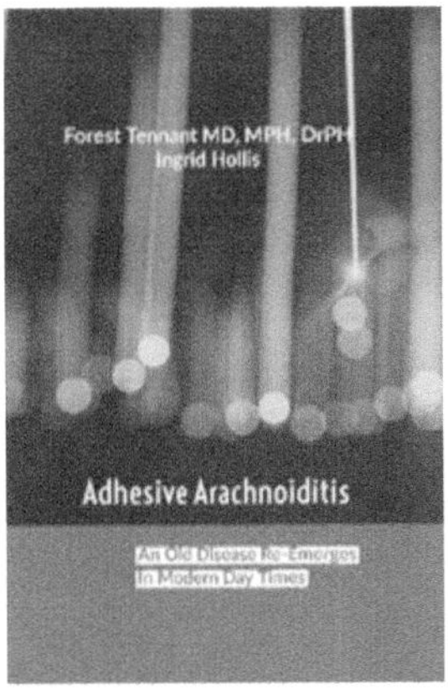

"ADHESIVE ARACHNOIDITIS: AN OLD
DISEASE RE-EMERGES IN MODERN TIMES"
ISBN: 9781955934039
LOC:2021912467

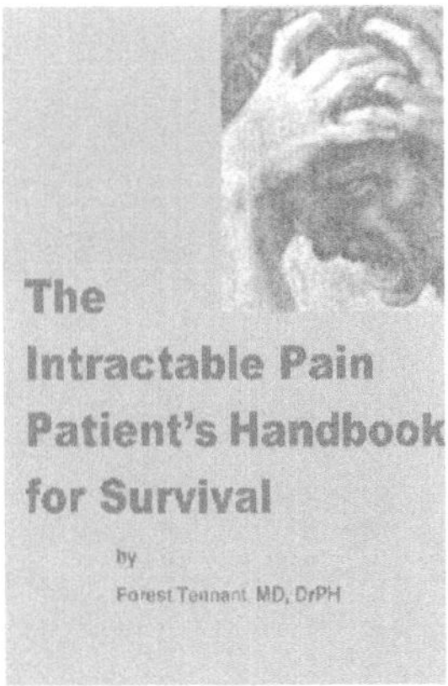

"INTRACTABLE PAIN PATIENT'S HANDBOOK
FOR SURVIVAL"

Tennant Foundation

Available on Amazon and where books are sold